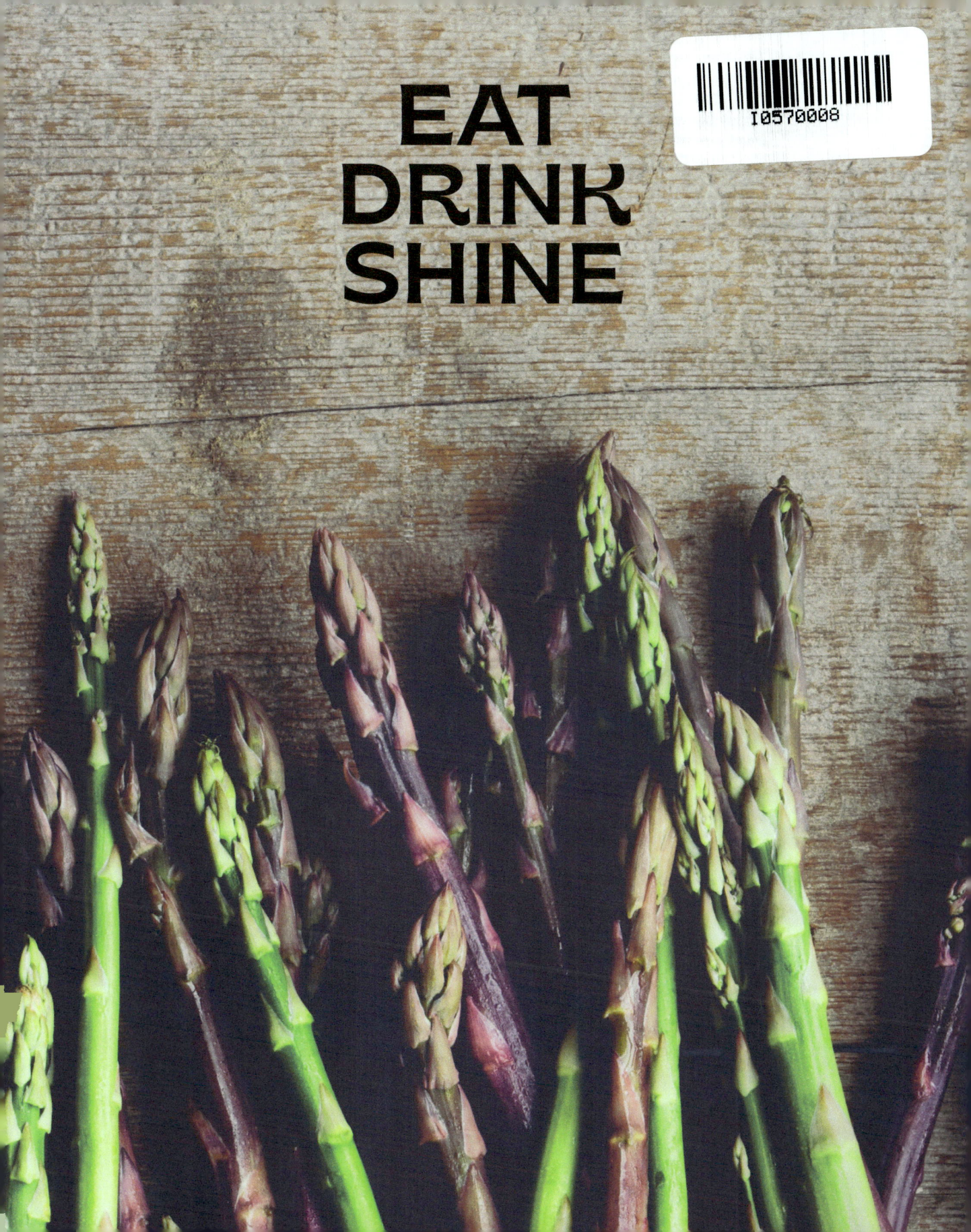

EAT
DRINK
SHINE

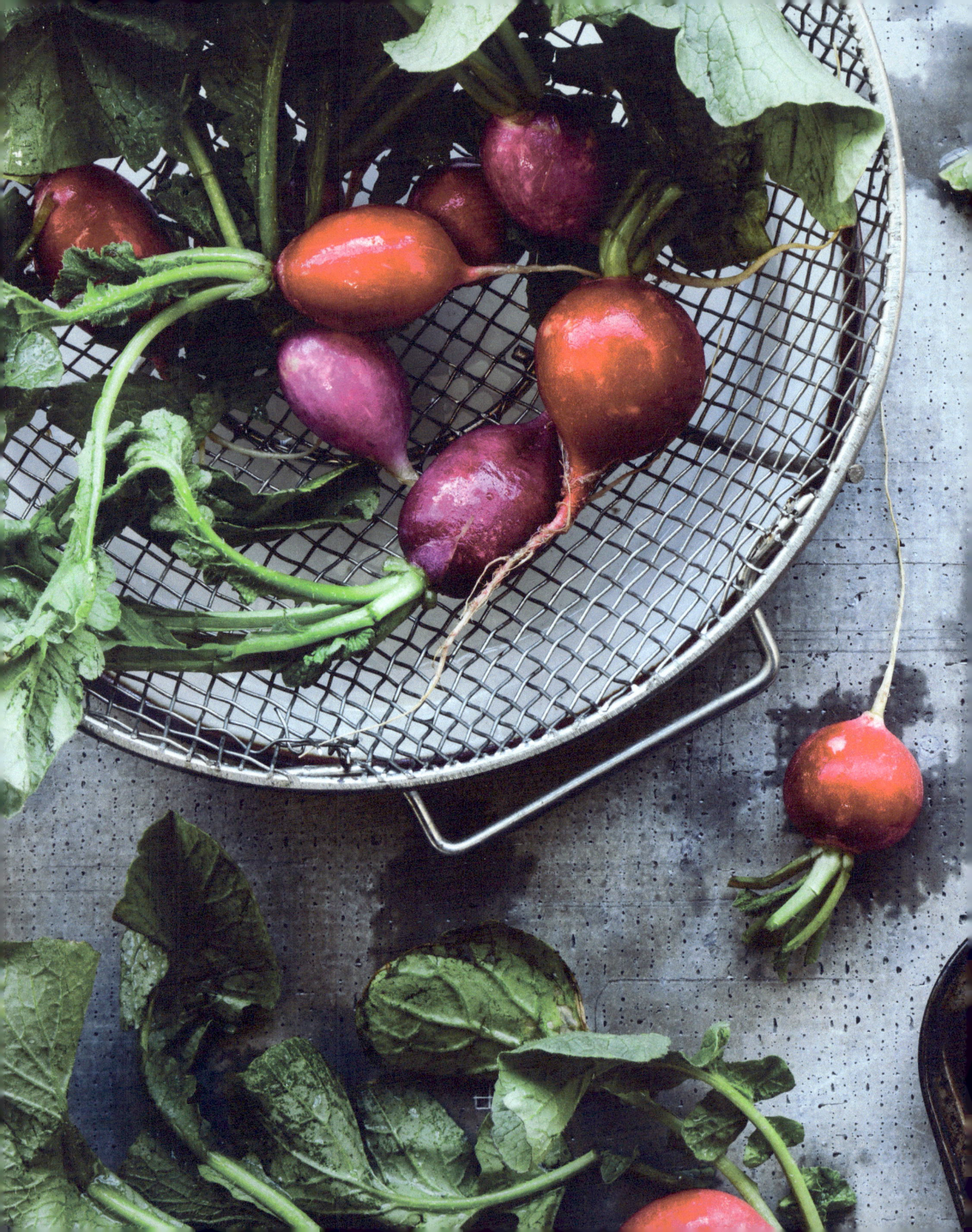

EAT
DRINK
SHINE

Gluten-free and
Paleo-Inspired Recipes

BY THE SHINE SISTERS
JESSICA, JILL & JENNIFER EMICH

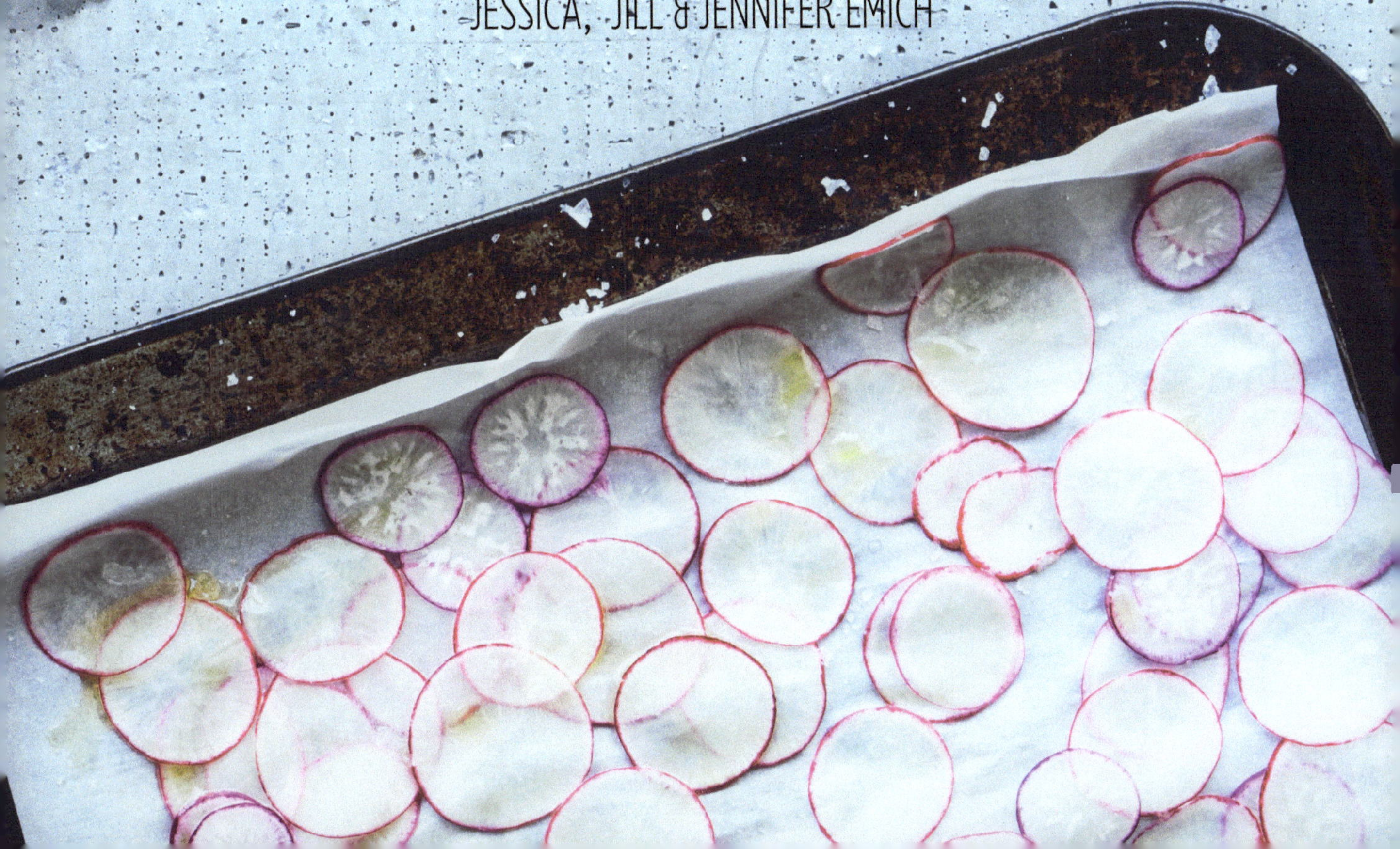

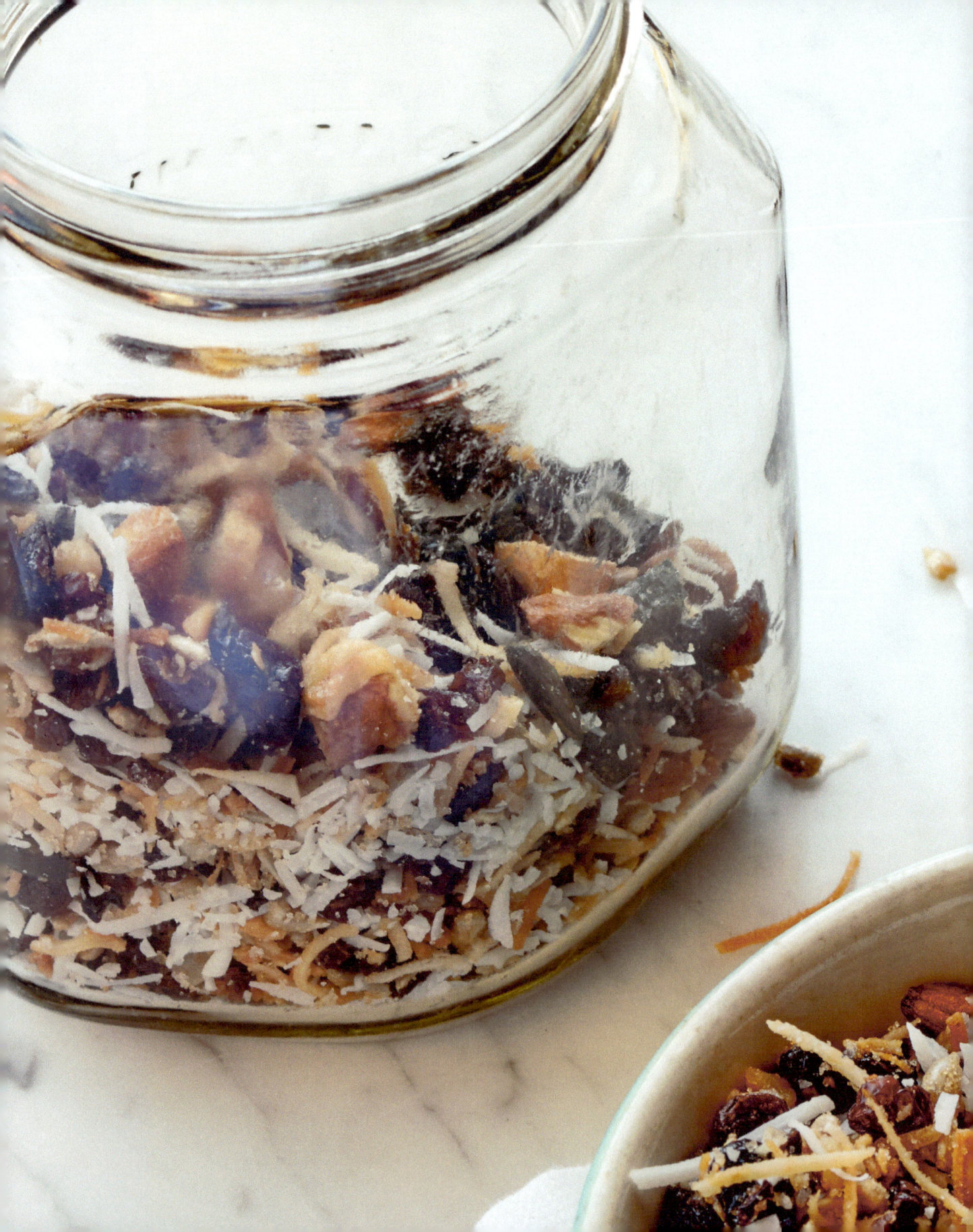

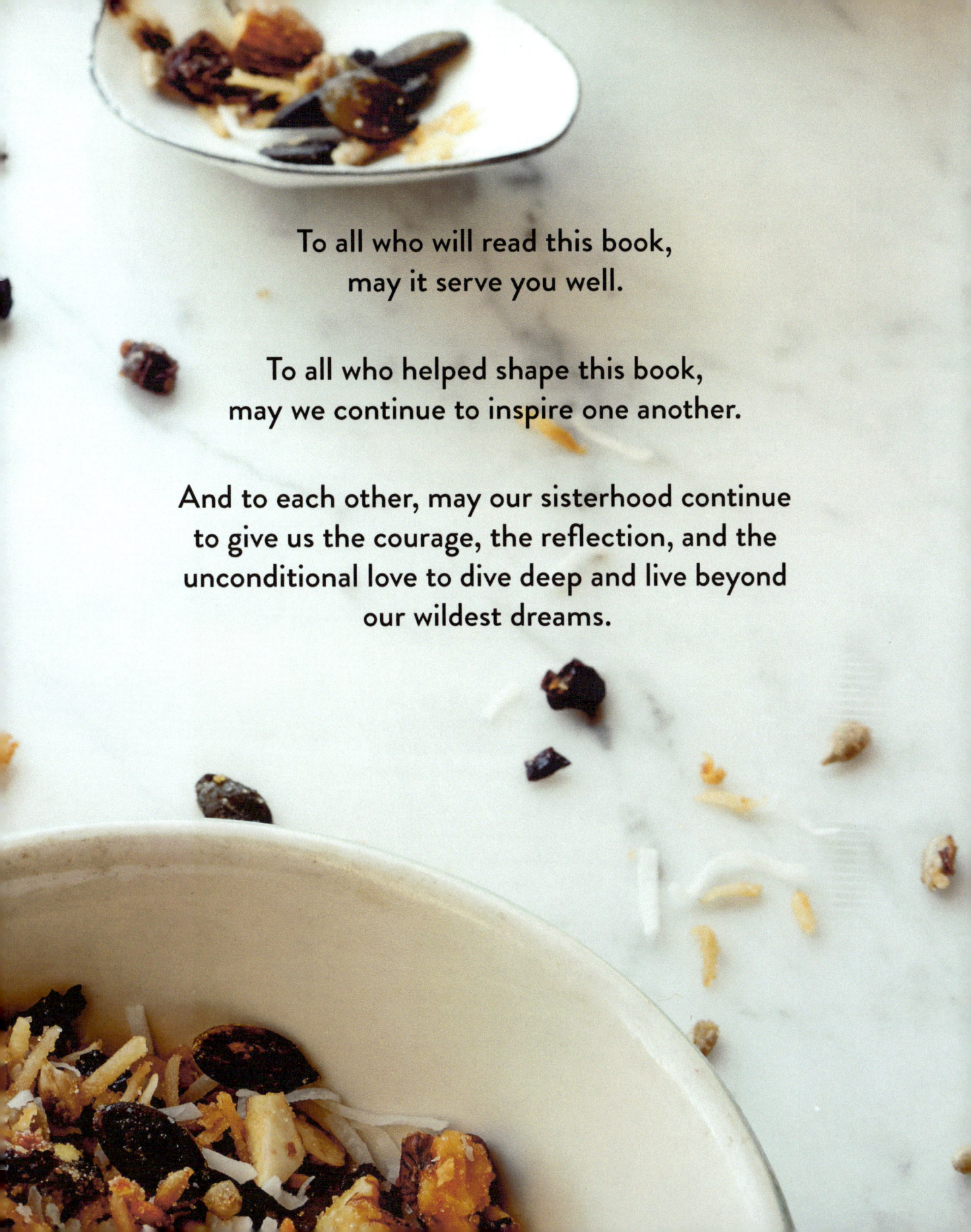

To all who will read this book,
may it serve you well.

To all who helped shape this book,
may we continue to inspire one another.

And to each other, may our sisterhood continue
to give us the courage, the reflection, and the
unconditional love to dive deep and live beyond
our wildest dreams.

Important note: The information and advice contained in this book are intended as a general guide to using plants and are not specific to individuals or their particular circumstances. Many plant substances, whether sold as foods or as medicines and used externally or internally, can cause an allergic reaction in some people. Neither the author nor the publishers can be held responsible for claims arising from the inappropriate use of any remedy or healing regime. Do not attempt self-diagnosis or self-treatment for serious or long-term conditions before consulting a medical professional or qualified practitioner. Do not undertake any self-treatment while taking other prescribed drugs or receiving therapy without first seeking professional guidance. Always seek medical advice if any symptoms persist.

Hardback ISBN: 978-1-956442-41-0
Paperback ISBN: 978-1-956442-42-7
Ebook ISBN: 978-1-956442-43-4
Library of Congress Control Number: Applied For.

Published by Highlander Press
501 W. University Pkwy, Ste. B2
Baltimore, MD 21210

Project Editor: Deborah Kevin
Designer: Catherine Williams | chapter-one-book-production.co.uk
Food Photographer: Eva Kolenko
Food Stylist: Jeffrey Larsen
Prop Stylist: Natasha Kolenko

SECOND EDITION

CONTENTS

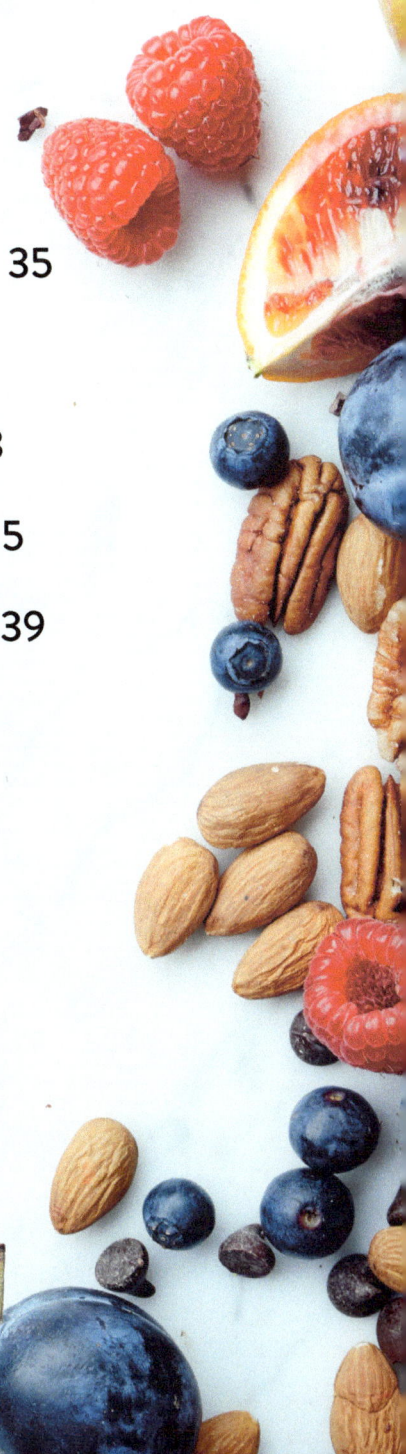

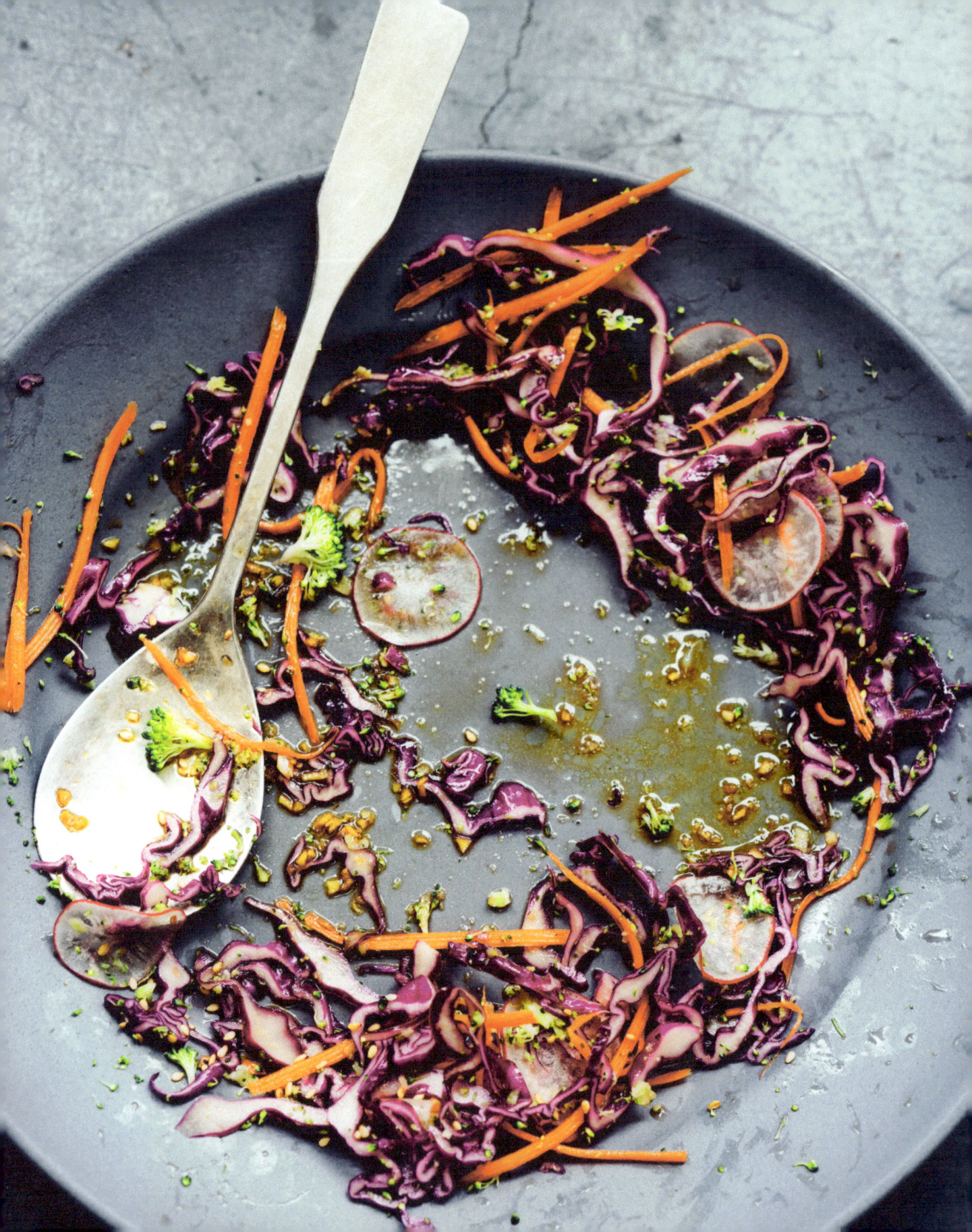

FOREWORD

I met Jessica, Jill, and Jennifer many years ago, while I was living in Costa Rica. Fresh out of high school and feeling unsure of what I wanted to do with my life, I decided to spend a few months traveling around Central America. Ten days into my trip I made it to Dominical, a sleepy surf town on the Pacific coast of the country. I fell madly in love with the place, and not having any responsibilities in life aside from making sure I didn't misplace my backpack, I decided to stay. I spent my first year immersing myself in the world of wellness. I started practicing yoga every day and would wake up at sunrise to meditate on the beach and then roll out my mat in one of the lifeguard towers, saluting the sun as it rose out of the jungle behind me. When I heard of a yoga retreat taking place in town, I decided to ask if I could join in. Jessica, Jill, and Jennifer, or the Blissful Sisters from Boulder as they were called, had teamed up with Wade Imre Morisette to lead a week-long retreat right around the corner from my house. This was the very beginning of my yoga practice, and never having taken part in a retreat before, I was unsure of what to expect. One of my earliest memories of my yoga practice is practicing with the triplets, being guided into Ardha Chandrasana, and falling over, while Jennifer was solid as a rock. I was filled with awe by her groundedness and calm and thought to myself; "one day I'll be that grounded, too."

The next day the sisters guided us through the world of food and nutrition. Having gone through so many changes in such a short time during my travels, my life was like a blank page. What did I want to fill my days with? What kind of patterns should I stick to when it came to my diet, and what should I drop? The sisters taught me so much about the connection between my well-being and the things I chose to fuel my body with throughout the day. This was the first time I had spent time contemplating the importance of eating real, whole foods from the earth. I was amazed by how different I felt when I chose to actually listen to my body. That one retreat with the Blissful Sisters was the beginning of a completely new life for me, a life where yoga, meditation, and nutritious foods together would become the foundation on which I built my life. It would still be years before I started teaching yoga, and I had no idea what life had in store for me at the time. Not in my wildest dreams could I have imagined that I would go on to lead my own retreats, write a New York Times bestseller, and dedicate my life to guiding people toward a balanced life in the future.

I am so grateful for having met Jessica, Jill, and Jennifer at the very beginning of my journey, and I know you are going to love this book just as much as I do. May it bring you lots of joy, nourishment, and inspiration in the kitchen!

Much love,

Rachel Brathen

Yoga Girl

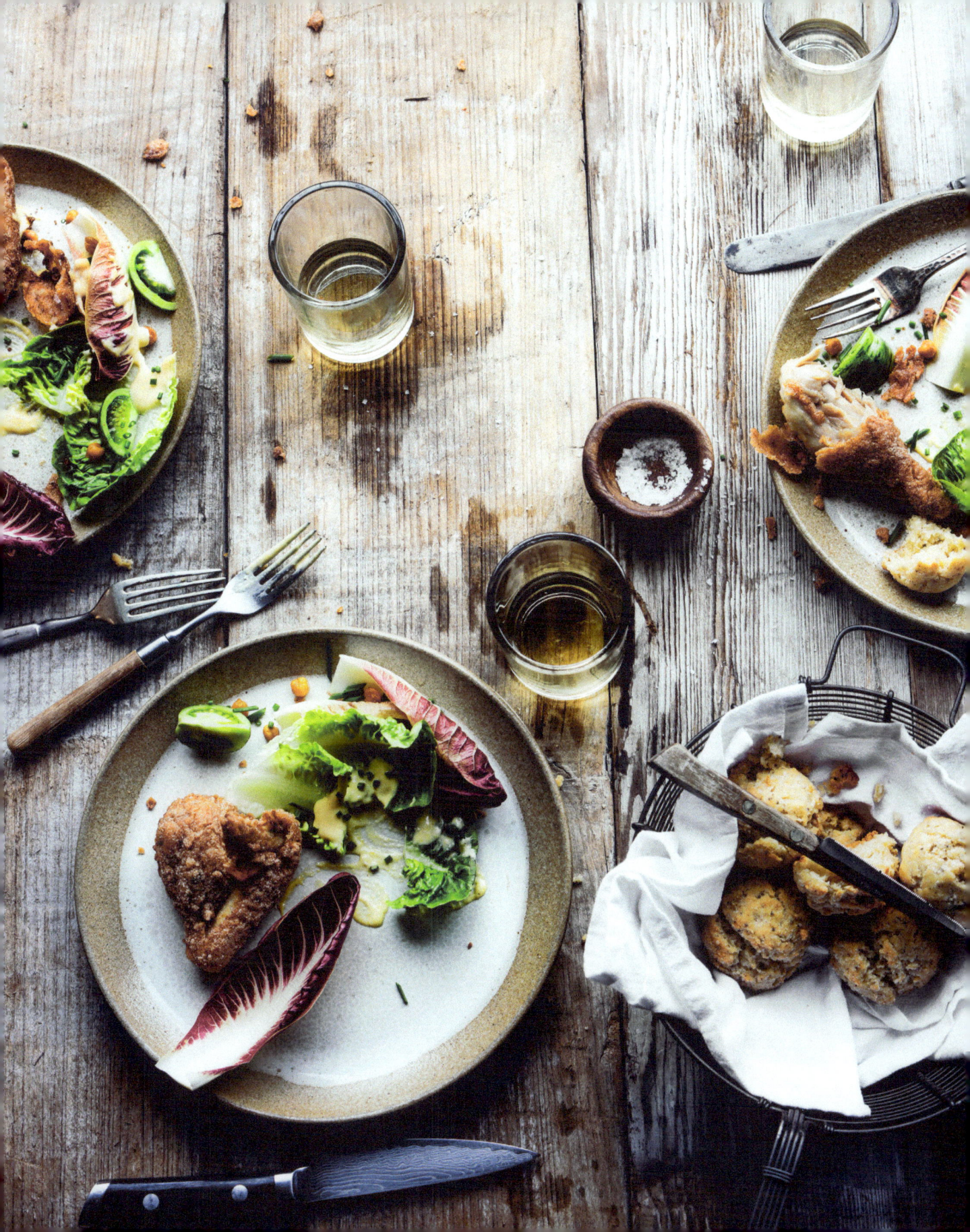

OUR STORY

Life is all about practice, trial, error, successes, and opportunities for growth. You never get to where you are going without first having to experience the journey, the wrong turns, the side paths, and the beautiful horizons. This book is not about preaching that there's one way, it's not saying that how we choose to live is the only way. We are all constantly evolving. Our intention is to inspire you to create a relationship with your body through your food, to listen deeply to it, to be at peace with your body, and to (dare we say it!) LOVE it. When you practice listening deeply to your unique body, it becomes less about others telling you what is right or wrong and more about feeling into what works for you. Your body is your home, it is where you reside—you can't move into another body or trade it in, you can only get to know it—what makes it tick, what lights it up and what makes it SHINE from the inside out. Food is a huge part of the experience.

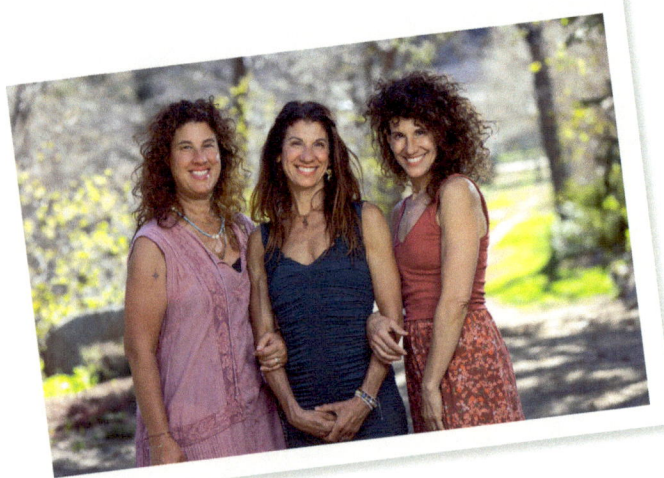

After owning restaurants for over twenty years, we have witnessed thousands of people and how they approach food. We have encountered people who have a fear of it, allergy and sensitivity issues of all kinds, and how we all can restrict ourselves. We have also witnessed how food can be a celebration, healing, transformative, and one of our greatest loves. The invitation is that you get real with yourself: how are you connecting with your

"YOU NEVER GET TO WHERE YOU ARE GOING WITHOUT FIRST HAVING TO EXPERIENCE THE JOURNEY, THE WRONG TURNS, THE SIDE PATHS, AND THE BEAUTIFUL HORIZONS."

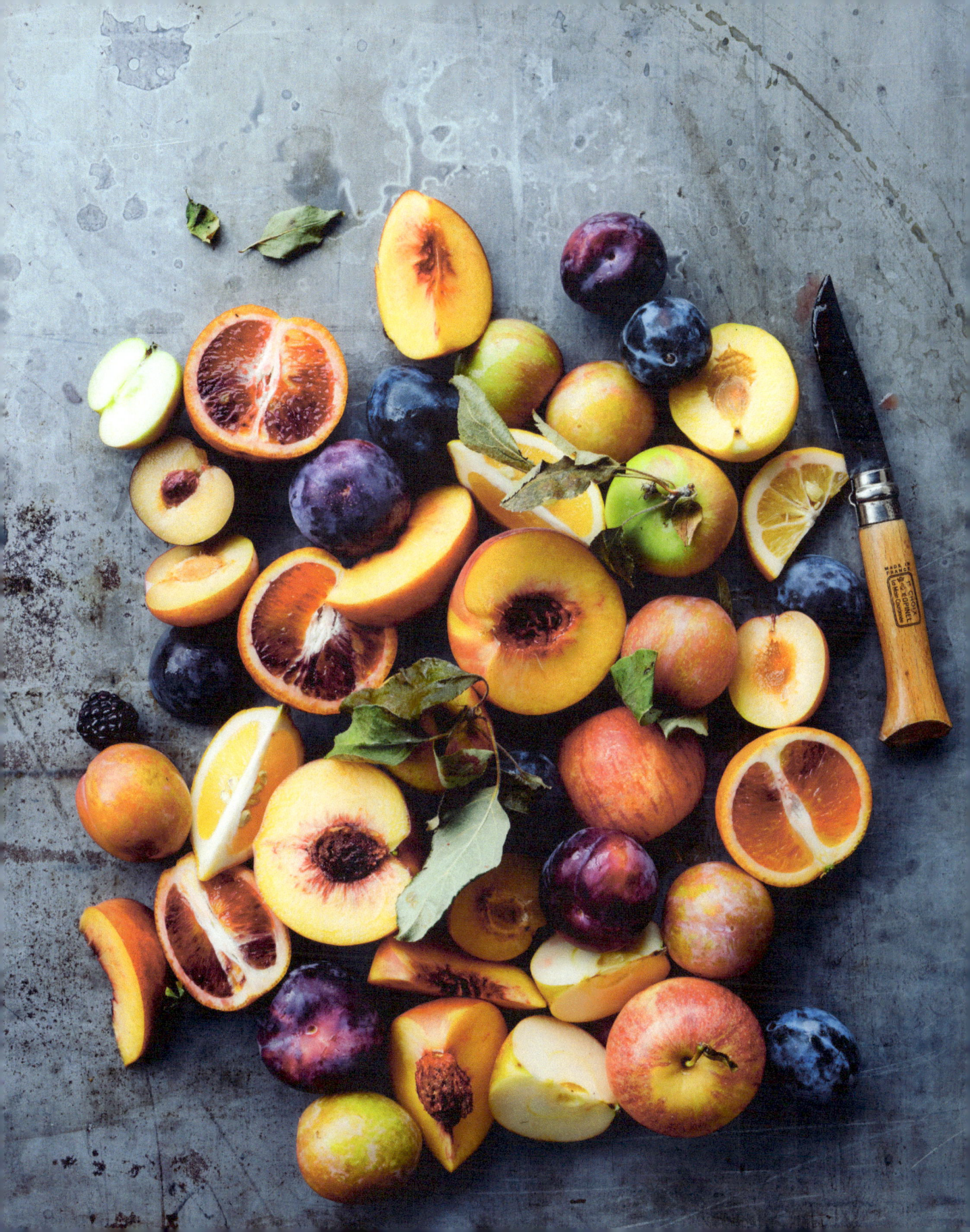

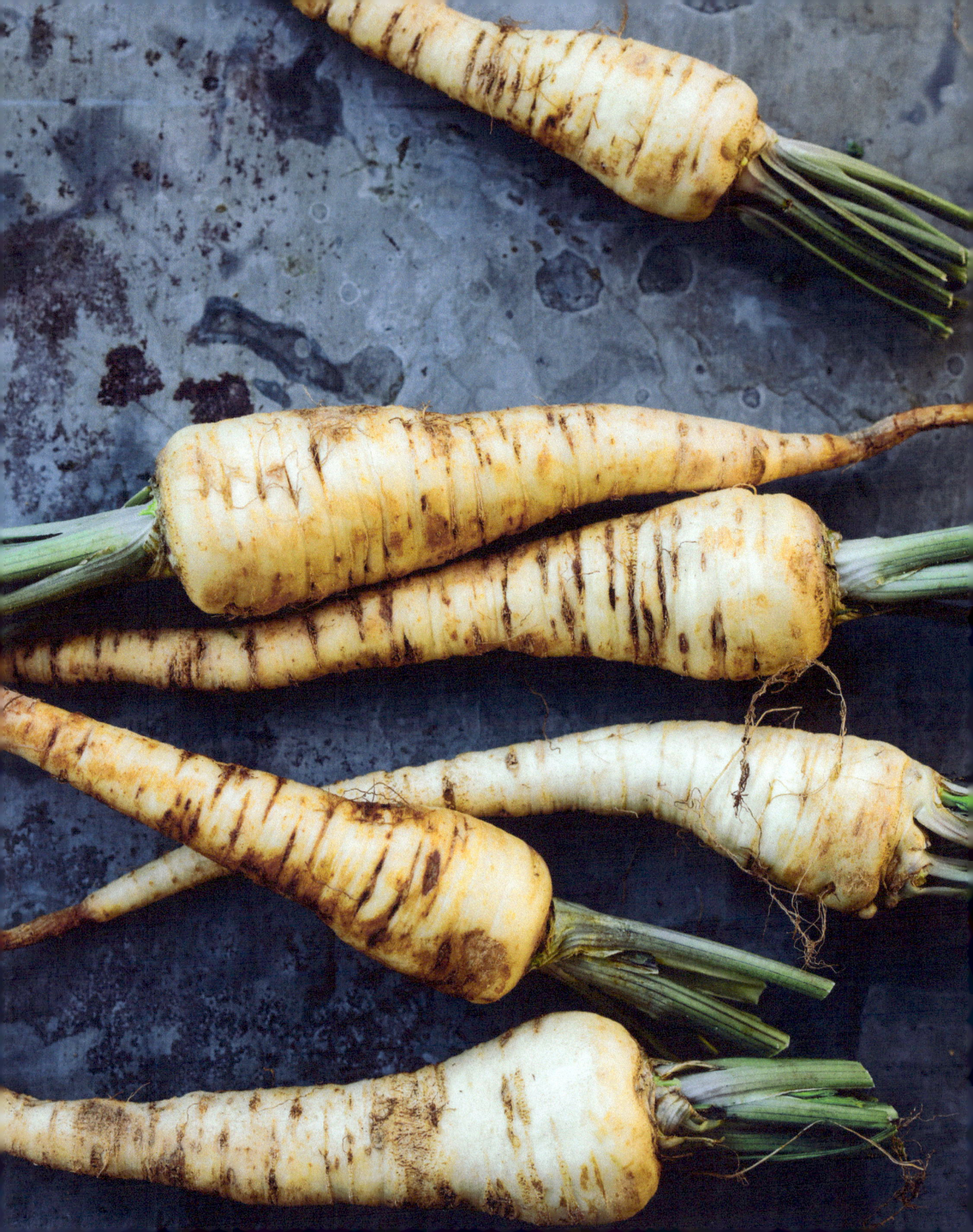

food, how does the food you eat make you feel? Once you understand the connection between how what you put into your body directly effects every single aspect of your life, we think you will understand how to EAT TO SHINE. For us it is the only way.

We are triplet sisters, yes, born on the same day four minutes apart from each other. We have been negotiating and navigating life with each other since the womb. Life together has had its amazing highs and devastating lows, but through it all, our connection to each other has been a constant source of love and support that has weathered every storm. We grew up in a huge Italian family where food was always a centerpiece of our lives, which is a large part of what drew us into the restaurant business and what stoked a desire to build a strong sense of community wherever we go.

Food gives life. Food is used in times of celebration and healing; it helps bring families and communities together. People fall in love and break up over meals. They laugh, cry, and have rituals around it. Food not only feeds our bodies, but also nourishes our souls and helps us radiate from the inside out. It is directly linked to our emotional well-being. We believe the relationship you have to food is very similar to the relationship you have with yourself and how you connect to the world. We all have to eat. So, we always say, why not enlighten ourselves and enjoy the ride. Our food literally becomes us. Everything we eat influences every cell of our bodies. And so, together we have made food our lives' passion.

"FOOD GIVES LIFE. FOOD IS USED IN TIMES OF CELEBRATION AND HEALING, AND IT HELPS BRING FAMILIES AND FRIENDSHIPS TOGETHER."

Together.... People always ask how it came to be that we chose to stay on a similar path all these years. In a sense, it wasn't a choice, it was our destiny. As little ones, our parents chose to dress us the same and even pinned nametags on each of our clothes! This led us to constantly strive for our individuality, but here we are writing a book together. We joked that it would break us as sisters, but this process has actually brought us closer together. It has been a beautiful journey that has deepened our relationship even further. As we get older, people are intrigued by us, three sisters who look alike, and the way in which we connect with each other. The unconditional love between us is palpable.

We come from a family where unconditional love, strength, patience, and compassion are woven throughout every nook and cranny of the household. Our older brother has a rare disease called Metachromatic Leukodystrophy. He is the glue of our family. He has taught us so much and has brought our family together in such a unique and fiercely loving way. Dennis has built a bond between us that will never go away. He has been a gift in that he has taught us to stick together even in the toughest of times. He taught us to look fear and the unknown straight in the eyes with love and trust. The life expectancy of his diagnosis was anywhere from 3 years to 25 years. Our brother is over 50 years old today and his doctors attribute his well-being over all this time directly to his care by his family. That means love and of course making sure he gets the nutrients he needs through his food. He is, for us, the ultimate lesson in how important family and inspired community is and that love truly does heal.

Our mom and dad have been married for over 50 years and have been so supportive of us and our wild roller-coaster lives over the years. We know it was no walk in the park to raise triplets on top of our brother and the extra care he needs. Growing up, our mom was a nurse on the graveyard shift in the intensive care unit in a New York City hospital and our dad was always working at least two jobs. But they never complained, they always were present for us, and they did more than make it work, they thrived with us and for us, and we are forever grateful. It is a gift that shines through in each and every one of our relationships.

But back to the food.... At age 11, we started working together in our uncle's grocery store. It was there that we started to understand food, to think about where it comes from, and the massive influence it has on every aspect of our existence. During our college years, we managed a restaurant together and it was a blast. We knew it was our calling to serve people in this way. Jessica and Jill went to culinary school after college while Jennifer spent time in Costa Rica teaching kids English. At the age of 24, we opened our first restaurant in Boulder, Colorado, and through our blood, sweat, tears, and laughter, food and community became our offering.

The restaurant was called Trilogy and it became iconic as a restaurant and nightlife scene for live music, partying, dancing, wining, and dining. It was a place where youth was explored and celebrated. There were late nights and wild times, and we loved every minute of it. It was inclusive, it was about community and connection, and about all walks of life communing over food, drink, music, art, and dance. After nine years we were good and fried and ready to move on. So, we sold it and moved on to individual projects, family, and our lives took their own paths. And then as it always does, a shift happened....

MEET THE SISTERS

Jennifer:

I met my husband Eck (Eric), a quirky, frenetic man from Connecticut, on a blind date in my 35th year. After seven months of dating , I was diagnosed with breast cancer , which was an absolute shock. The night before my test results came back positive, Eck got down on one knee and asked me to marry him regardless of the outcome. It was the single most profound experience of my life. He committed to walking this path with me and my family even though we were still getting to know each other. It has been 14 years and the journey of a lifetime, both the marriage and fully healing from cancer through food and continuing to find ways to harness joy and gratitude no matter what. It taught me that we truly are our own healers on so many levels. Post restaurant, I followed in my family's footsteps as a now third-generation woman realtor and real estate investor. I love continuing my passion for bringing joy to others and learning and growing within myself.

Jessica:

Running restaurant kitchens for almost twenty years was quite the undertaking for me. It is a high-energy and sometimes stressful environment, but I loved it. It became a wonderful practice for me to access inner calm amidst the chaos. It is a skill that will serve me for the rest of my life. Having earned a master's degree in Holistic Nutrition, it has always been my mission to create food that is deeply nourishing as I know how vital health-giving food is to both physical and emotional health. After the restaurants, this mission continues as I nurture my daughters and husband and our community with nutritionally inspired recipes. My passion for health and wellness is central to my life. That is why we created Shine Living Community, where I teach yoga, meditation, nutrition, and cooking. I love that we bring kids into the practices at Shine Living Community. In today's world, with so much technology and social media influence, I find it so powerful to lead the kids back to their hearts and their unique gifts and to remember how powerful they are. And, of course, they teach us! They remind us to connect with our own inner child. I am amazed at how powerful it is to practice and play together.

Jill:

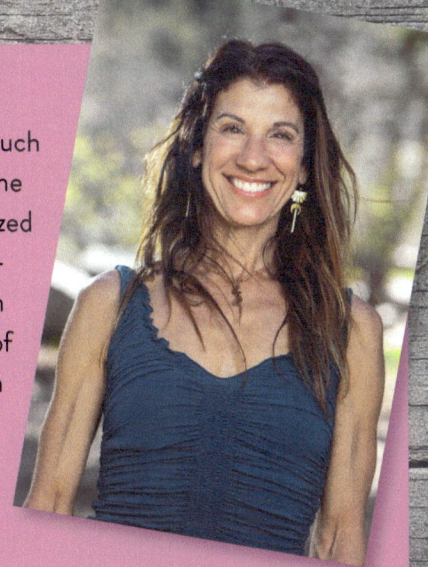

In my twenty-three years of owning and running restaurants, I learned much about nourishing people through food, community, and self-love. After the Trilogy days, I was still single and flailing in that department. I finally realized I was a chronic people pleaser, and although it worked great in the restaurant, not so much in intimate relationships. I realized I needed to focus on what "I" wanted instead of giving away what I thought the other wanted of me. But at that point, I wasn't even sure what that was. Between the high stakes and busy and joyous world of running our restaurants, I started solo expeditions around the country and beyond, which was an edge for me. In the edgy parts, I found myself, I found my strength, and I practiced loving myself through it all.

At forty-two, I became a dance instructor and choreographer. I then completed a program to become a Somatic Therapy coach and mentor. I became a certified Breathwork instructor. I blended all of these modalities together, plus my unique imprint, and I taught, led, and learned in new ways. I love it so much.

In 2022, my sis Jessica and I created Shine Living Community—a global community to do this work of finding self and uplifting the whole through movement medicine, grounding practices, and delicious food; together in community, it has been an incredible ride. Oh, and the guy... as soon as I got to the place of self-love and a deeper understanding of what I wanted, he came in. When I looked into his eyes, I knew I had found home. I met Steve when I was forty-two, and we were married shortly after. For my entire journey that is still unfolding, I am forever grateful. So, now, my mission in life is to continue to dig deep within, learn, grow, and invite others to do so, too.

Back together again... we opened a second and third restaurant, Shine Restaurant & Gathering Place and Shine Restaurant & Potion Bar. We also launched one of the first woman owned breweries in the country, Shine Brewery and an herbal beverage company, Shine Potions. After a culmination of 23 years, a pandemic and new dreams in our hearts, we decided to spread our wings beyond the four walls. This book is by family for family, and not just brothers, sisters, parents, and children, but family meaning all of us everywhere. All of our recipes have a celebratory feel because we believe in the kind of food that makes you feel good. We use pure ingredients, holistic techniques, and recipes that are great for sharing. For the past 20-plus years, we have been feeding others through our nourishing restaurants and gatherings. Now is the time to extend our offering to you!

From the heart,

The Shine Sisters

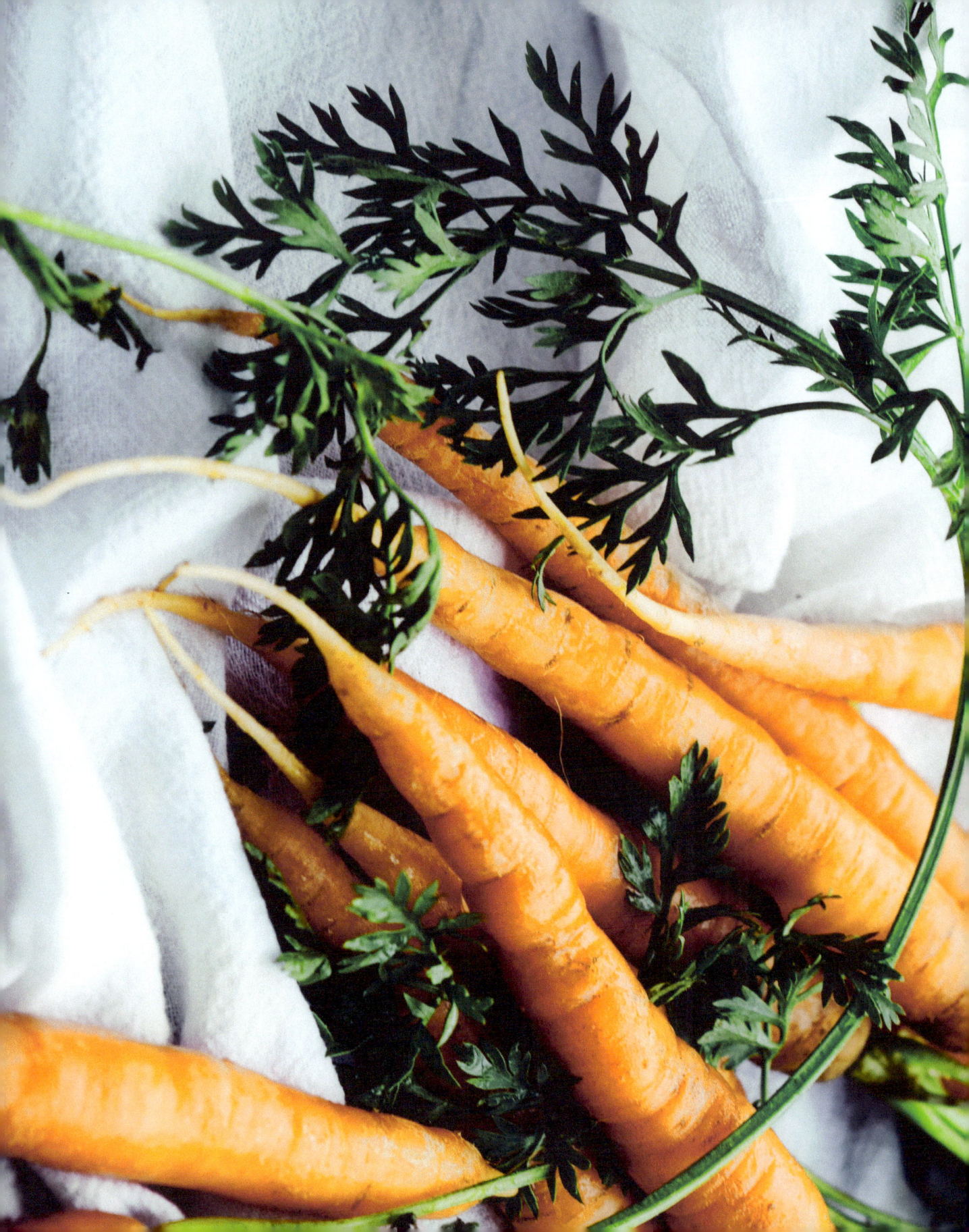

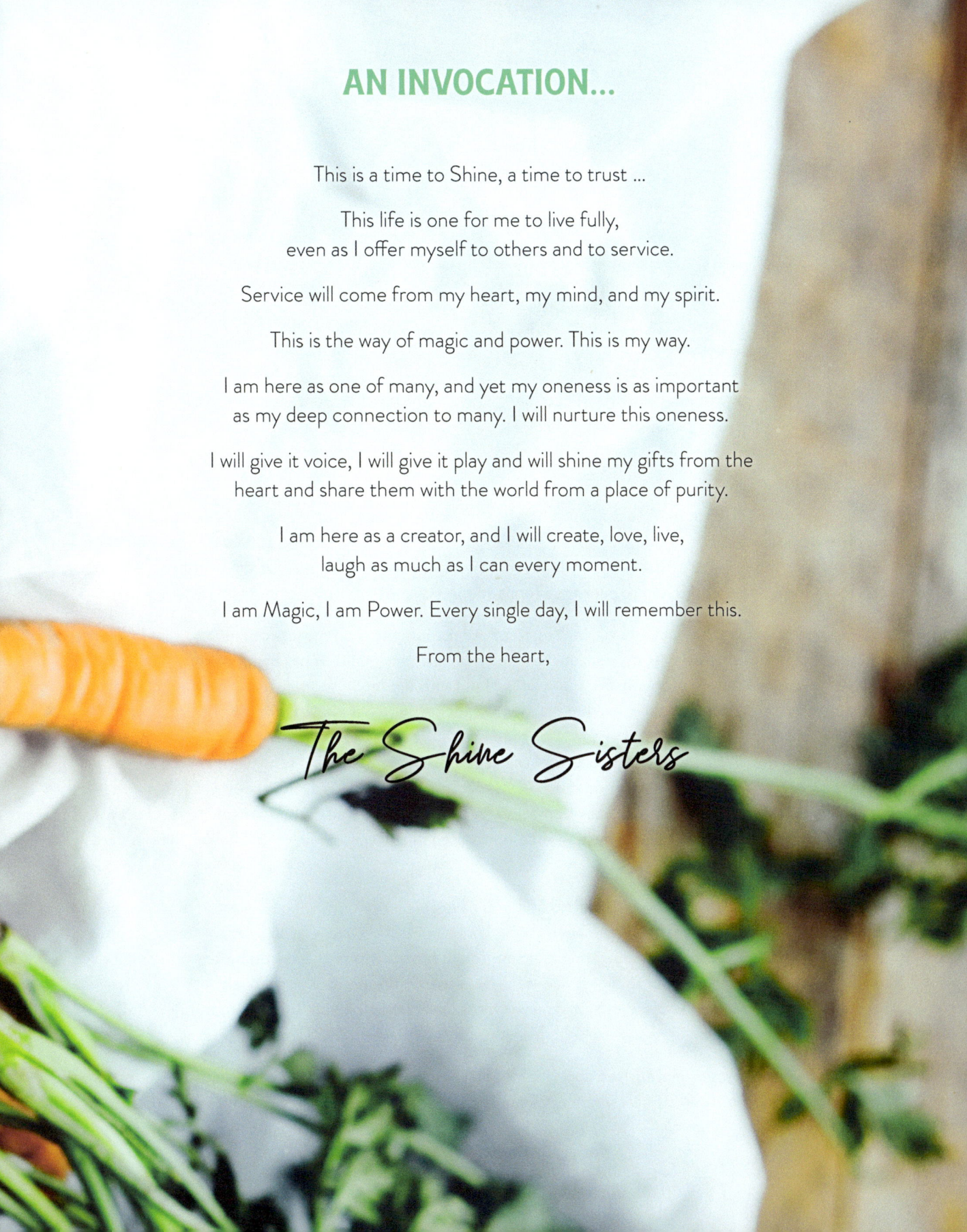

AN INVOCATION...

This is a time to Shine, a time to trust ...

This life is one for me to live fully,
even as I offer myself to others and to service.

Service will come from my heart, my mind, and my spirit.

This is the way of magic and power. This is my way.

I am here as one of many, and yet my oneness is as important
as my deep connection to many. I will nurture this oneness.

I will give it voice, I will give it play and will shine my gifts from the
heart and share them with the world from a place of purity.

I am here as a creator, and I will create, love, live,
laugh as much as I can every moment.

I am Magic, I am Power. Every single day, I will remember this.

From the heart,

The Shine Sisters

THE GLORY OF GLUTEN-FREE AND PRAISE FOR PALEO

Jennifer: Growing up, I had a serious case of psoriasis. Parts of my skin would get itchy and scaly, and I almost always had a sporadic rash. I would feel congested and sneezy. Eventually the straw that broke the camel's back was a full-body rash, and I knew I needed to get control of what was happening. I took a blood test and it came back positive for a gluten intolerance. I cut gluten out of my diet 15 years ago and have never had another skin reaction. Although my sisters don't have the same sensitivity, they have chosen to eat gluten in moderation and they feel the benefits.

Gluten is a protein found in many grains such as wheat, semolina, spelt, kamut, rye, and barley. It is a protein that gives bread and dough its fluffy texture and chewy nature. It's also used as a stabilizing agent in many processed foods, such as salad dressings and mayonnaise. It keeps them from separating or "breaking." It's in everything from beauty products to packaged foods to medications and supplements.

Gluten on its own is actually not the villain. Yes, it is harder to digest than most proteins, and that in itself may be difficult for some people, but really what it comes down to is, gluten has been overprocessed and therefore it has caused problems for many of us. Gluten is hidden in so many processed foods. A lot of times, it is eaten at every meal in excess. Also, wheat, barley, and oats have often been sprayed with chemicals, and then refined and processed until they are barely recognizable by the body and therefore hard to break down. We believe that because of this it caused many issues like sensitivities and allergies to gluten. The fact that we are eating too much of it, that it is overprocessed, and that it is a protein that is harder to digest than most other proteins creates a perfect storm. As a result, a sensitivity started to develop in many people. If people's digestion is compromised in any way, they will most likely have a hard time digesting gluten.

Gluten is best eaten in moderation regardless of if you have an allergy or not. The digestion of gluten can be supported by eating it in foods that have been through a fermentation process, such as soaking glutenous grains overnight before cooking or by eating it in sourdough breads where the fermentation process breaks down the gluten, making it easier to digest. Celiac disease is a different story. Individuals with celiac are not able to tolerate gluten in their diet at all and will most likely never be able to tolerate it. For them, gluten-free is a way of life.

We have chosen to create a gluten-free cookbook as well as a gluten-free restaurant because, after working in the food industry for over 20 years, we have found that many people are having issues with gluten.

We have seen through our experience that going gluten-free will help heal the gut and create a stronger digestive fire, which translates into more energy and stronger health overall. We have chosen to create a gluten-free cookbook as well as a gluten-free restaurant because, after working in the food industry for over 20 years, we have found that many people are having issues with gluten. We have seen through our experience that going gluten-free will help heal the gut and create a stronger digestive fire, which translates into more energy and stronger health overall.

Paleo is eating close to the earth, in a way that's very similar to how our ancestors ate before the industrial age. It is, in a nutshell, eating whole unprocessed foods like grass-fed meats, free-range chicken, wild fish, lots of fresh vegetables, natural fats, and nuts and seeds while eliminating grains, legumes, and limiting dairy, unless it is raw dairy. It is cutting out foods that lead to inflammation in the body. It is said by many who have switched to this way of eating and now even an increasing number of doctors and nutritionists that the Paleo way of eating is energizing and brings you to your body's natural and healthiest weight. It is simple, clean, easy to digest, healing, and wholesome. It means eating a healthy balance of fats, proteins, and carbohydrates in a culture that is inundated with processed, overly starchy, and added-sugar foods.

What we like about this way of eating is that it is a framework that can be tailored to individual needs, depending on your sensitivities, genetics, and desires. Our bottom line is to listen to your body and see how a variety of foods make you feel. If you know your digestion is off, your energy levels wane, or you have skin irritations, it is worth switching things up, experimenting with a Paleo and Gluten Free way of eating, and seeing if you experience positive changes. Your inner fire is everything. If you feel energized and inspired, life is a playground and you can engage in a playful manner.

The recipes in this book are 100-percent gluten-free and Paleo-inspired. We are 80/20s, meaning we eat Paleo about 80 percent of the time, so we've shared some of our favorite nutritious non-Paleo dishes with you as well.

About the Recipe Icons

DF Dairy-free

PI Paleo-inspired

V Vegetarian

All recipes in the book are gluten-free

Jill: I am pretty active in my life and exercise almost every day, including teaching dance, Freedom Movement classes with my sis, or filming for our online digital studio, Shine Living Community. What I love about the paleo way of eating is that a big part of it is the quality of ingredients, with a focus on wild meats, organic local vegetables, and whole foods. I am not strict, but I am dedicated because this way of eating gives me plenty of energy, and I feel clear and focused throughout my day. I also love supporting local farms, and because my husband is a reverent hunter, we enjoy wild Colorado game often. I have had the honor of learning to prepare every part of the animal.

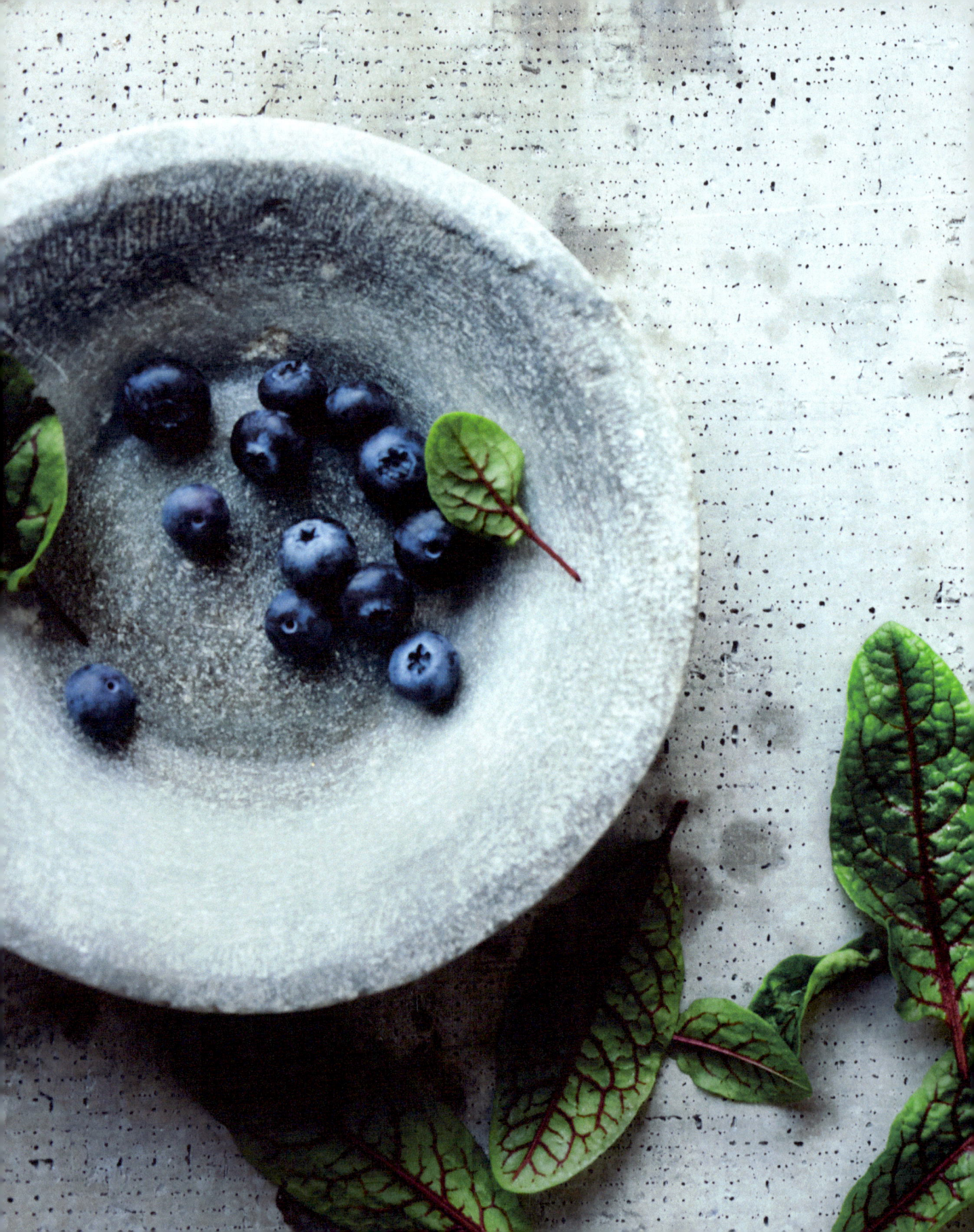

WAKE UP & SHINE

Every morning we get to begin again. Your morning sets the tone for the rest of the day. We love fueling up on a wholesome breakfast to feed the body, brain, and spirit. These recipes are easy, fulfilling, and will get your tank, aka your glorious body, properly filled. Reset, Ready, and Go.

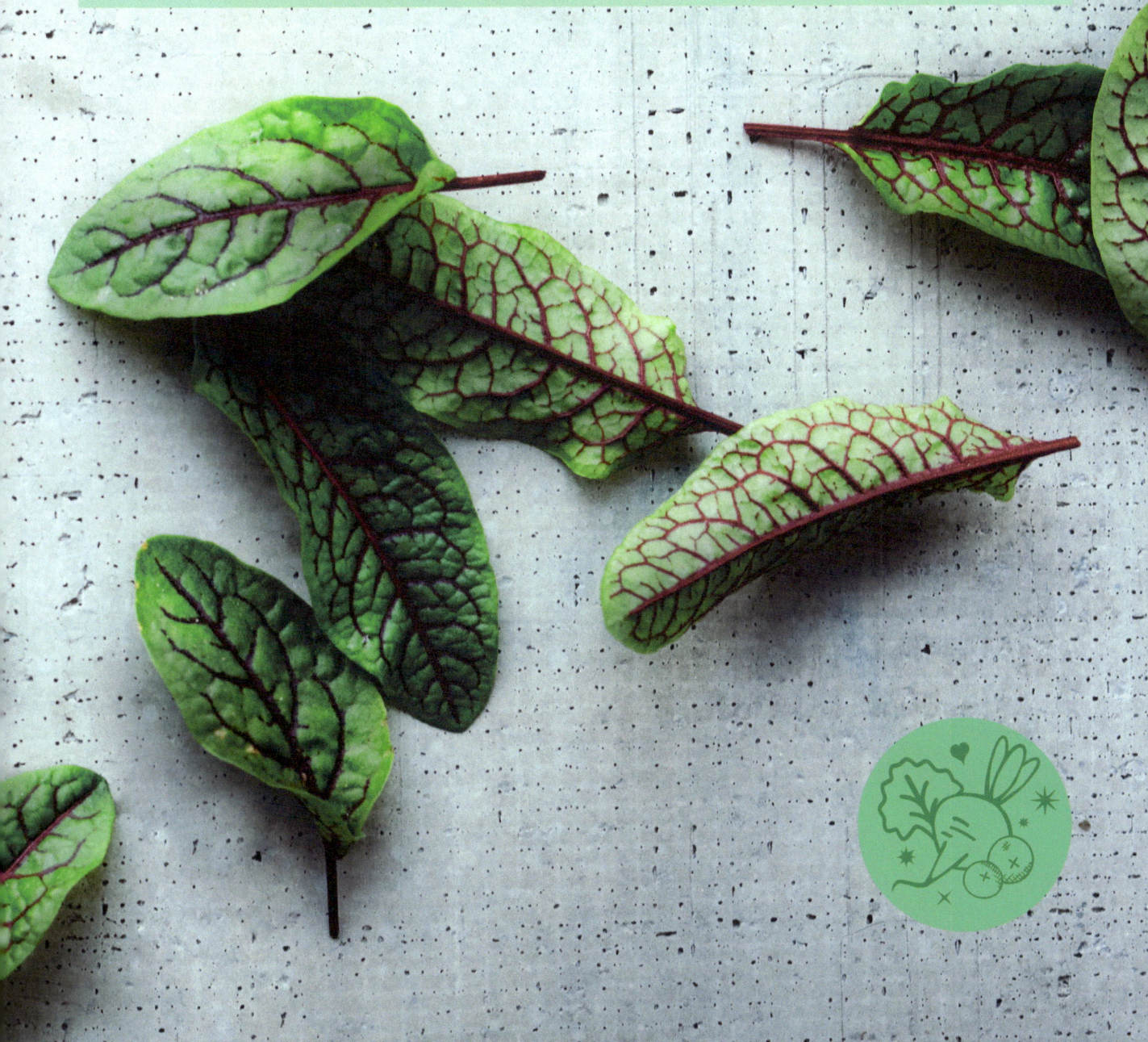

BEGIN WITHIN

Get Your Game On:
Morning Routines by the Shine Sisters

Jill Emich shares her Morning Routine to start the day in her SHINE avatar. Read on for eight powerful tips and a sugar scrub recipe, too.

I like to say that every day, we get to begin again. Forget New Year's Resolutions. Let go of the guilt of being hard on yourself for something you wish you didn't do yesterday. How about this: every morning your body awakens is a chance to reset. And I believe how you start your day sets the stage for what you attract into your life. The curtain goes up—there is a motley cast of characters, whether it be your kids, your co-workers, or the person driving behind you—and they are all part of the plotline. Every day will be full of revelations, lessons, and growth.

You never know exactly where a day will take you, but you can set yourself up for success by getting in the right mind- and heart-set through movement and nutrition.

Here are some of my favorite morning practices:

1. *Give Thanks.* I wake up with gratitude for a new day and that I get to choose how I want to interact with the world. I think of three things I am grateful for—first thing.

2. *Drink Water.* I mix warm water with lemon or lime and a sprinkle of sea salt. I use two mugs or a 16-ounce mason jar. This not only starts my body off hydrated and kicks my metabolism into gear, but it also aids digestion, is an anti-inflammatory, and boosts the immune system. I drink before any stimulants like green tea, mate, or coffee.

3. *Exercise.* Whether it is fifteen minutes or an hour, I leave some time to get my heart rate up most days. One of our Shine Living Community workouts takes less than fifteen minutes and leaves me PUMPED. Then, if I am sitting in front of my computer, I don't feel as much tension or body aches. (Note: if I DO have to sit in front of my computer for the majority of the day, about every hour, I get up and either take a walk outside for a few minutes or just take a walk around the building to keep the blood flowing. I find if I do this, I stay motivated, and my brain stays in the game).

4. *Quiet Time.* A breathwork and meditation practice that allows me to check in with how my emotional and physical body is feeling and use my breath to balance and ignite my system. If there is any anxiety in any part of my body, I sit, put my hands over it, and focus on breathing there and allowing it to release. Three minutes can do the trick.

5. *Caffeination.* Coffee, mate, or green tea: I mix it up! I try not to have it when I awaken; my caffeine intake happens after quiet time and exercise, which helps me avoid becoming addicted to caffeine to wake up first thing in the morning. I want to ensure my body remembers that it doesn't need caffeine to be active.

6. *Blend a Smoothie.* I make a smoothie with greens, spirulina, flax seeds, MCT or coconut oil, blueberries, or a banana. These good fats, protein, fiber, minerals, and vitamins give me a nutrition and energy boost that will last all day and keep me satiated until early afternoon.

7. *Detoxify the Skin.* I make my own scrubs to use in the shower, which leaves my skin feeling soft and helps with detoxification. Some basic exfoliating gloves (a dry brush works well, too).

8. *Set the Mood.* I turn up some tunes while I get ready to go. You might catch me dancing to one of my favorite songs I choreographed. I wear clothes that are comfortable and feel good on my skin. I head out the door feeling juiced, ready for the curtain call. Bring it, life; this girl is READY.

Jennifer:

I love to wake up early enough in the morning to get some quiet time in. It is my time to get my head clear, check in with my heart, and set forth on the right foot. I drink warm water with lemon to aid the digestive system; it's a cleansing and detoxifying way to start the day. Most mornings I have our pressed green juice (page 149) to give me a natural energy boost instead of caffeine. I do love the flavor of coffee and tea, but I try to wake my body up through food first and have caffeine in the later part of the morning.

After my daily beverage ritual, I move my body. I love walking and hiking outside or doing yoga. It is too easy for me to hop on my computer in the morning, but I try to get in at least 30 minutes of exercise beforehand, so I can feel more energized and grounded throughout the rest of the day. I feel so blessed to live in a place where the sun shines most days. Living at a high altitude, in a sunny state, I make sure to stay well-hydrated. Making it a top priority to get movement daily helps my body and mind be in optimal health, so I can make sure I am in tiptop shape to handle all the curveballs, staff, and guests that I am surrounded by at Shine every day.

Jessica:

Two of the things I love to do in the morning before the kids get up is move and meditate. Even if I am headed out to the mountains or to teach a Freedom Movement class later in the morning, this intentional movement to get things flowing sets the tone for the day. Also, sitting with my Beingness in a quiet meditation has been a game changer for my emotional health and clarity of the path ahead.

We have created the Warrior Workout Method, which I practice first thing in the morning. I wear my headphones to assure I get this time to myself and not draw attention to the kids.

The Warrior Workout How-To:

- Put on music that makes you want to move. We love tribal drumming for this.

- For about 3 minutes, start shaking along with mini jumps like you are shaking it up and shaking it off because you are! This should get your heart pumping and every part of your body jiggling and moving.

- Root your feet and start dynamic movements. For example, twists in the spine or switching back and forth, lifting each knee, arching your back, bending forward, circling your neck, or circling the torso—whatever your body is asking for.

- End by standing still and closing your eyes, feeling the roots of your feet sink into the earth, your heart soft and open, and the center of your head expanding while breathing long, slow breaths up and down your spine.

- Feel into your primal nature and connect with the energy you created in your body.

SHINE SUGAR SCRUB

I like mainly using sugar as it moisturizes the skin, but I add about a quarter cup of Epsom salts for extra detoxification. Ensure the granules are small so they don't scratch the skin. I use ¾ cup melted coconut oil and ¼ cup sesame oil for added vitamin E and anti-aging benefits. You can also use olive oil or sweet almond oil. The basic blend is one-part oil to two-parts sugar/salt. I also add a few drops of my favorite essential oils. Mix in a bowl with a spoon and store in a glass container. You can make it in 10 minutes and keep it in a jar in the shower. This scrub turns your shower into a spa treatment!

SOFT-BOILED EGGS

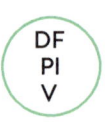

DF
PI
V

Our mom is the master of the soft-boiled egg. It always felt so good to wake up to warm eggs that we could scoop right out of the shell. Just add a touch of sea salt, a dollop of ghee, and it's instant satisfaction. We love serving them with a side of cooked greens for a balanced power breakfast.

Serves 2

2 large eggs
Avocado Mash
(page 23) or Avocado
Hollandaise (below),
for serving (optional)

1. Put the cold eggs in a small saucepan and cover them with cold water. Bring to a boil. Turn off the heat, cover the pot, and let sit for approximately 5 minutes (see Tip).

2. To eat your egg, crack the top with a back of a spoon and peel away enough shell so you can insert your spoon to scoop out the egg. Serve with avocado mash or avocado hollandaise, if you like.

TIP

The size and temperature of your eggs will have an effect on your timing. This is something to pay attention to so you can get consistent results every time.

AVOCADO HOLLANDAISE

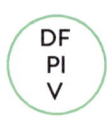

DF
PI
V

The avocado in our "hollandaise" sauce helps it taste rich and decadent, with a smooth consistency, even though it is egg and dairy free. It is easy to make and our guests at Shine go bonkers for this alternative to the classic topping for poached eggs. We also love it as a topping for greens, fish, or rice, as a dipping sauce for veggies, and as a spread on a sandwich.

Makes about 1 cup

1 ripe avocado
1 tablespoon fresh
lemon juice
2 teaspoons chopped
fresh dill
1 teaspoon hot sauce
½ cup extra-virgin olive oil
Sea salt to taste

Cut the avocado in half lengthwise. Remove the pit and scoop out the avocado flesh into a food processor or high-powered blender. Process the avocado for 30 seconds or so, then add the lemon juice, dill, and hot sauce and pulse two or three times. Slowly drizzle in the oil and process for another minute until smooth and pourable. If the sauce is too thick, then add some water, a tablespoon at a time, until the desired consistency is achieved. Season with salt just before serving.

TIP

This is best made the same day you are using it for maximum flavor and freshness.

PERFECTLY POACHED EGGS WITH AVOCADO HOLLANDAISE

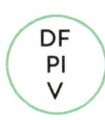

Served on top of our Cured Salmon and drizzled with Avocado Hollandaise, our Perfectly Poached Eggs make an Omega-3-packed power breakfast or brunch—the perfect alternative to classic Eggs Benedict. We also like them on their own, with some Avocado Mash alongside.

Serves 2

2 large eggs

Avocado Mash (page 23)

Sea salt to taste

Avocado Hollandaise (recipe opposite)

1. Fill a small saucepan with about 4 inches of water. Bring the water to a boil and then reduce the heat to a low simmer.

2. Carefully crack each egg into a separate small bowl (careful not to break the yolks!). One at a time, very gently tip the bowls so that each egg falls into the simmering water. With a spoon, push aside any whites so they don't run into each other. Cover with a lid and turn off the heat. Your perfect poached egg will be ready in 5 to 7 minutes (see Tip for cooking times by preference).

3. Season with sea salt, drizzle with the avocado hollandaise, and serve immediately.

TIP

Poaching preferences:
5 minutes for soft
6 minutes for medium
7 minutes for hard

BAKED EGGS IN AVOCADO CUPS

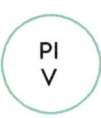

This is a breakfast high in protein and great fats to make you energized as you step into your day. Smaller eggs are better to use than large ones here, as the flavor is more concentrated and they will fit better in the avocado cups. For an extra kick and added protein, serve with our Cultured Salsa (page 46) and a sprinkling of chopped bacon.

Serves 2 to 4

2 ripe avocados

4 small farm-fresh eggs

1 tablespoon ghee (page 24) or unsalted butter, melted

Sea salt to taste

1. Preheat the oven to 400°F.

2. Cut the avocados in half lengthwise and remove the pits. Using a tablespoon, scoop out 1 to 2 tablespoons of avocado flesh from each half to create 4 cups, each large enough to hold one of your eggs. (This is a delicate process that will result in the ideal results if the eggs are on the small size. Size matters here.)

3. Crack an egg into each avocado "cup." Yolks first followed by the whites if room allows. Drizzle each with the melted ghee and sprinkle with sea salt.

4. Arrange the avocado cups in a small baking pan to fit them as close and snug as possible. Bake for 15 to 17 minutes, until the egg whites look cooked through. Serve immediately.

TIP

If you have left over avocado you can rub the flesh lightly with a few drops of lemon and olive oil and cover tightly with plastic wrap to keep the freshness and make the color last longer. Best if eaten within a day or two.

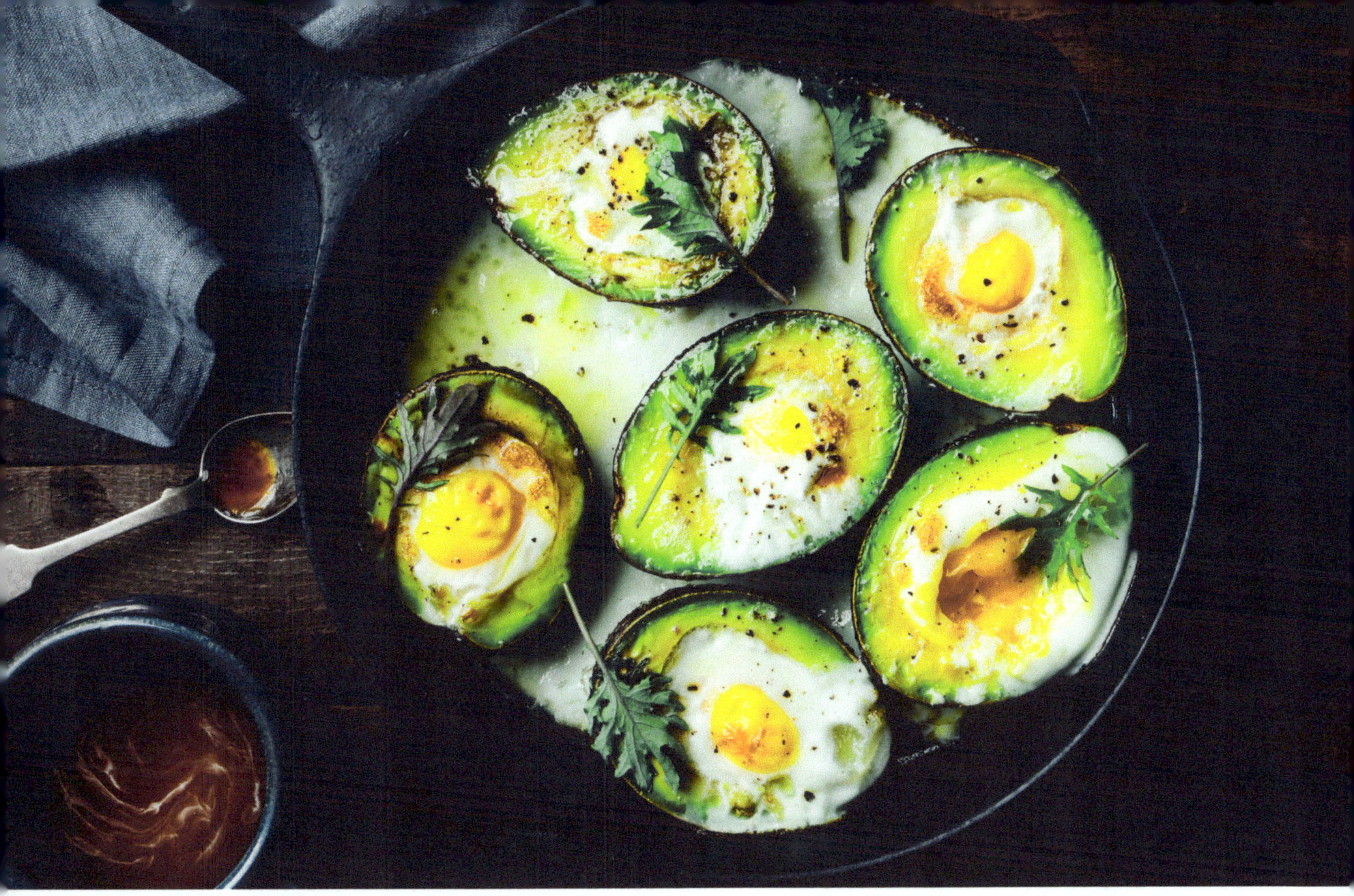

AVOCADO MASH

Avocados are a superfood. They equalize blood sugar and cholesterol. Avocados are loaded with heart-healthy monounsaturated fatty acids and fiber to keep your system moving. They are a fantastic fat to incorporate into your daily diet. We serve this mash alongside our Cured Salmon (above), spread it on toast, or use it as a dip.

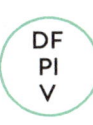

DF
PI
V

Makes about 1½ cups

2 ripe avocados

2 teaspoons finely chopped red onion

½ teaspoon minced garlic

1 teaspoon apple cider vinegar

sea salt to taste

1. Cut the avocados in half lengthwise, remove the pits, and spoon out the flesh into a large bowl. Lightly mash the avocados with the back of a fork.

2. Add the red onion, garlic, and vinegar to the bowl and mix together. Season with salt. Serve immediately.

TIP

This mash can be made into more of a guacamole-style dip if you add 2 to 3 tablespoons fresh lime juice and 1 heaping tablespoon freshly chopped cilantro..

Jill: Ghee is butter with the milk solids removed. It has wonderous health benefits. I add it to coffee (see our Root to Rise Coffee, page 155) and smoothies and love to cook with it. It is much more stable for high-heat cooking than regular butter and many oils because it has a higher smoke point, so it's less likely for your kitchen to get smoky when you're pan-frying or sautéing in ghee. It actually has a more buttery flavor than plain butter and much more nutritional value as well. Some people that have a hard time digesting dairy can actually eat ghee. I love the smell when it is simmering on the stovetop. I am all about the ghee. I use it generously daily.

HOMEMADE GHEE

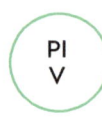

PI
V

Makes 3 cups
2 pounds chilled unsalted butter, grass-fed when possible, cut into small cubes

1. Gather the following tools together to make your homemade ghee: a small bowl, small strainer, sterilized 1-quart glass jar, and several pieces of cheesecloth for straining the butter.

2. Melt the butter in a pot over medium heat. When it's fully melted, let the butter come to a light simmer, then reduce the heat to low-medium (see Tip). A thick foam will start to form on the top. Continue to simmer as the foam first increases, then decreases and dissipates as the milk solids begin to attach to the sides and the bottom of the pot. Allow the solids to sink to the bottom, lightly scrape the sides of the pot with a silicone spatula to assist.

3. Continue to scrape the sides of the pot so the solids do not burn. After 5 to 7 minutes, the butter will start to clear as the milk solids begin to brown at the bottom of the pot. Turn off the heat once the butter begins to lightly foam again.

4. Allow the butter to cool slightly and the foam to settle, then strain the ghee through the cheesecloth into the sterilized glass jar.

5. Stored in the jar at room temperature, your ghee will keep for 2 to 4 months.

TIP

It is important to cook the butter over low to medium heat to help the milk solids separate. We have found that doing this too low and too slowly sometimes create a murky product in the end instead of the clear ghee we desire.

AMARANTH PORRIDGE

Soaking whole grains, legumes, and nuts is an important step before eating these foods. They contain a coating that protects them in nature, but also makes them challenging to digest as well as making some of their nutritional value unavailable. Soaking these foods for 6 hours or overnight dissolves this coating and creates an easy-to-digest, highly nutritional food. We soak all grains, nuts, and legumes for the restaurant. It is a challenge to do this in a high-volume restaurant, but we wouldn't have it any other way.

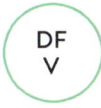

DF
V

Makes 5 cups or 4 to 6 servings

2½ cups full-fat canned coconut milk

2 cups water

2 cups amaranth, soaked overnight, drained, and rinsed

2 teaspoons vanilla extract

½ cup maple syrup

½ teaspoon ground cinnamon

1. Pour 2 cups of the coconut milk and the water into a medium pot and bring to a boil. Add the amaranth and return to boil. Reduce the heat to a simmer and cook for 20 minutes.

2. Add the remaining ½ cup coconut milk and mix well. Return the heat to medium-low and cook another 10 minutes, until most of the liquid has absorbed and the amaranth is tender.

3. Remove from the heat and stir in the vanilla and maple syrup. Sprinkle with the cinnamon (do not mix it in yet), cover the pot, and let the porridge stand for 5 minutes before serving. Refrigerate leftovers in an airtight container for up to 1 week.

TIP

This porridge is delicious topped with a variety of nuts or berries, sliced banana, or a spoonful of ghee. It is a perfect recipe to make in advance so it's ready to just heat up in the mornings.

Jill: After an early morning dance session on the beach at our family beach house, as I walked up to the house, I witnessed my mother spoon-feeding my brother this porridge. I sat and watched them. They were in silence, but there was so much love passing between them. When I went inside, my mom said to me, "I just love taking care of him." It was a beautiful statement about unconditional love that's emblematic of what this porridge means to me... comfort and security. When we were kids, my mom made farina as a warm and comforting breakfast. This is our family's latest hot cereal made with amaranth, an ancient gluten-free grain that is dense with minerals and has more protein than most other grains. The maple in place of the white sugar we used to use adds additional minerals and just the right sweetness.

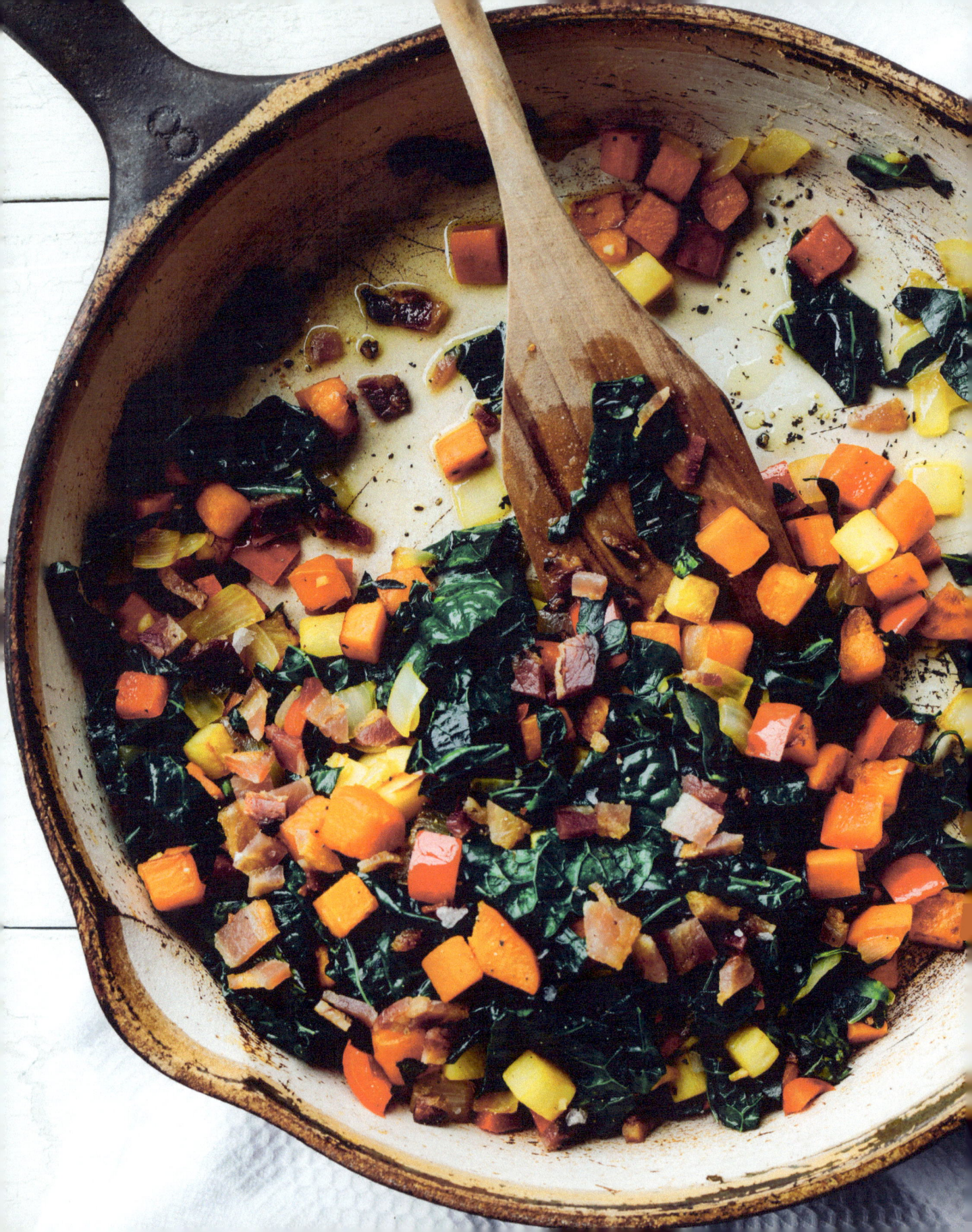

SWEET POTATO AND KALE HASH

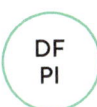

DF
PI

This hash can be a side dish or main, paired with eggs or Cured Salmon (page 28), or both. We like it because it is fast to make, easy to clean up (only one pan required), and an enjoyable way to get a hefty dose of veggies. You can switch up the vegetables to use up whatever you have in your refrigerator.

Serves 4 to 6

2 strips uncooked bacon (optional)

1 tablespoon coconut oil or ghee (to make your own, see page 24), plus more if needed

1¼ cups diced or grated sweet potato

¾ cup diced assorted root vegetables (we love carrots and turnips here)

½ cup diced bell pepper

¼ cup diced onion

1 small bunch kale, destemmed and chopped into bite-sized pieces

1 teaspoon minced garlic

Sea salt to taste

1. Cook the bacon, if using, in a large sauté pan over medium-high heat, until crispy on both sides. (No oil is necessary as the bacon will render its own fat.) Remove from the pan and let cool, leaving the fat in the pan.

2. Melt the coconut oil in the pan (use only ½ tablespoon if you rendered the bacon in the pan). Add the sweet potatoes and root vegetables to the pan and sauté until mostly tender, 7 to 10 minutes. Add the bell pepper and onion and cook another 5 minutes. Add the kale and garlic and sauté for approximately 1 minute. Season with salt and cook another 3 to 5 minutes. (If your hash becomes dry or begins to stick to the pan, add another tablespoon of coconut oil.)

3. When all the vegetables are tender and the flavors have commingled, turn off the heat and add the reserved crispy bacon, if using. Serve hot.

TIP

Add cooked ground grass-fed beef or ground turkey to make this hash a hearty one-pan meal.

CURED SALMON

It is important to use wild salmon in this recipe to get the benefit of higher Omega-3s, which support health benefits including heart health, healthy cholesterol levels, and optimal brain function. In addition, wild has more flavor and a better texture. Ocean pollutants are also much more concentrated in most farmed fish. There are exceptions with sustainable farming methods, so talk to your local fish guy or gal to find out which seafoods are the best choices. We like to serve this with Avocado Mash (page 23) on toast, with eggs, or in Sweet Potato Hash (page 27). Note: this recipe takes three days to cure, so plan accordingly!

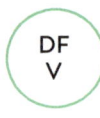

Makes 2 pounds

2 (1-pound) salmon fillets, skin on, deboned, pin bones removed

1 cup sea salt

½ cup sugar

10 sprigs or ½ ounce fresh dill

Avocado Mash (page 23; optional)

1. Rinse the salmon under cold water and pat dry completely with paper towels. Combine the salt and sugar in a small bowl.

2. Lay out the fillets, skin sides down, on a cutting board or clean work surface. Pour the salt and sugar mixture onto the flesh, dividing it evenly between the fillets, and rub it in. Top each fillet with half of the dill sprigs.

3. Lay one piece of salmon on top of the other, with the pink fleshy parts of the fillets facing each other. Make sure you sandwich the dill in there nicely.

4. Tightly wrap the entire salmon "sandwich" in plastic and put it in a shallow nonreactive container. Cover the salmon with more plastic wrap. Top with something flat (a small clean cutting board is perfect) and weigh the salmon down with a heavy can.

5. Refrigerate for 3 days, flipping the salmon sandwich over every 12 hours or so. Make sure to drain and discard any accumulated liquids and reposition the weight on top of the salmon each time.

6. After 3 days, unwrap the salmon, thoroughly rinse it with water to remove all of the salt and sugar, and pat it dry, keeping the two fillets sandwiched together.

7. To serve, very thinly slice the cured salmon, cutting only as much as you plan to use. Serve with avocado mash alongside, if you choose. Wrap the rest of the fillet sandwich whole in plastic and refrigerate on a plate or in an airtight container. The cured salmon will keep for 2 to 3 weeks.

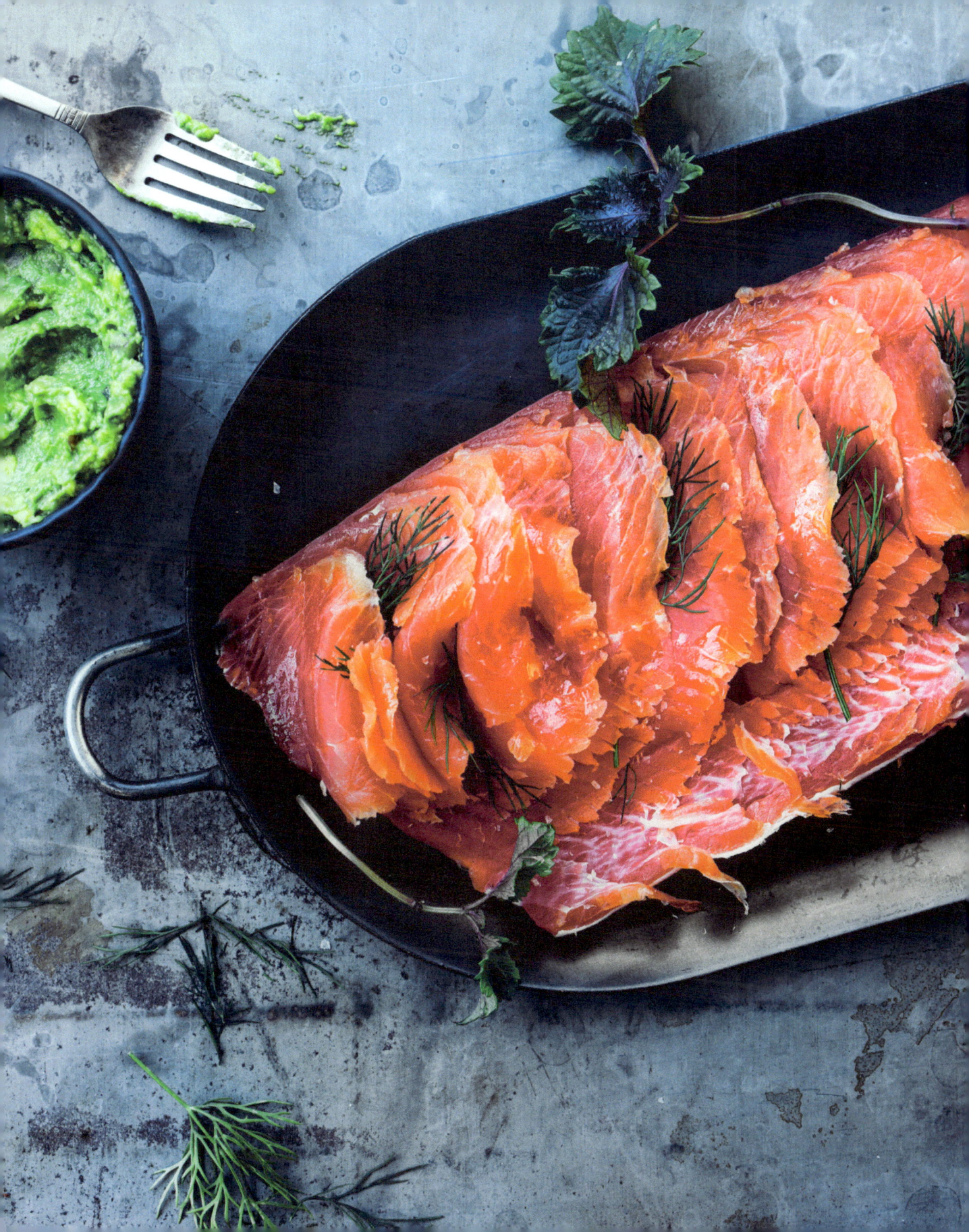

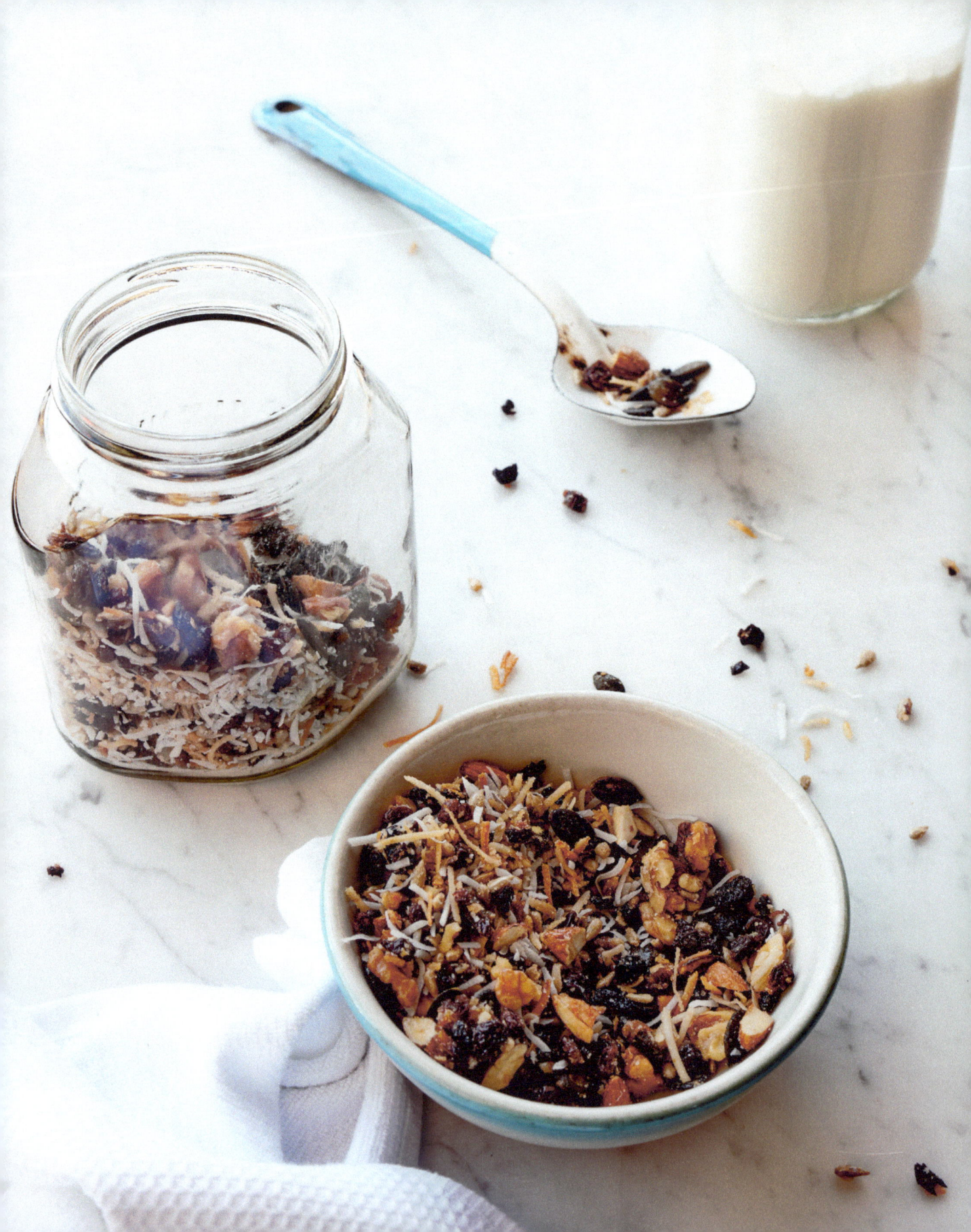

RAW PALEO SPROUTED GRANOLA

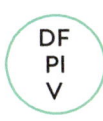

DF
PI
V

This sprouted granola may sound like a lot of work, but it is worth it! Actually, most of the time that goes into this recipe is for the dehydrating process. It keeps for at least 2 months and makes a big batch so you prepare it once and enjoy it for a long time. Serve with milk or yogurt—or eat it alone as a trail mix. Just be warned: it can be addicting!

Makes one (64-ounce) mason jar or four pounds

1 cup raw shelled sunflower seeds

1 cup raw shelled pumpkin seeds

¾ cup raw walnuts, chopped

¾ cup raw almonds, chopped

1 cup dried cherries, chopped

1 cup raisins, chopped

8 dried dates, chopped (Medjool variety is delicious)

1½ cups raw coconut flakes

½ cup maple syrup

2 teaspoons vanilla extract (to make your own, see page 171)

2 teaspoons sea salt

½ cup coconut oil

1. Thoroughly wash and rinse all of the nuts and seeds. Combine in a bowl, cover with filtered water, and let soak at room temperature overnight.

2. The next morning, drain and thoroughly rinse the seeds and nuts. Spread them out on dehydrator trays and dehydrate at 105°F (or on the seed and nut setting on your dehydrator). This will take 6 to 8 hours, depending on your dehydrator. (If you do not own a dehydrator, see Tip.)

3. Transfer the dehydrated nuts and seeds to large bowl and toss with the dried cherries, raisins, dates, and flaked coconut. Add the maple syrup, vanilla, and salt, mixing thoroughly to coat.

4. Heat a large pan or pot on low heat. Add the coconut oil and let melt (this takes 1 to 2 minutes). Add the nut and dried fruit mixture to the coconut oil. Toss several times to coat, then remove from heat.

5. Lay out parchment paper on two baking sheets or on the kitchen counter. Pour half of the granola mixture onto each sheet of paper, spreading it out evenly. Let harden overnight.

6. In the morning, mix the granola one more time with your hands. It will last for up to 2 months stored in a glass container in the pantry.

TIP

You can also dry out the nuts and seeds at a low temperature in the oven. Arrange them on a baking sheet and place them in a low oven (about 115°F) for at least 4 hours or overnight until they are completely dried and crisp. If you are concerned about keeping the nuts raw, it is important to maintain the 115°F temperature.

SHINE'S BUTTERMILK BISCUITS

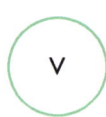

Our guests go crazy for these gluten-free biscuits, which have always had a cult following at the restaurant. One of our chefs, Nelson, created the recipe, which we serve with eggs or as a dipper for soups and stews, and even as a decadent sandwich bread.

Makes 16 small biscuits

½ cup plus 2 tablespoons (¾ stick) unsalted butter

1 cup tapioca flour

½ cup brown rice flour

½ cup millet flour

½ teaspoon xanthan gum

1 teaspoon sea salt

1½ teaspoons baking powder

1 tablespoon chia seed (optional)

1 cup buttermilk

1. Cut the butter into 1/2-inch cubes and place in the freezer to chill for at least 10 minutes.

2. In a bowl, whisk together together the three flours, the xanthan gum, salt, baking powder, and chia seed, if using. Transfer to a food processor. Add the frozen butter and pulse 15 to 20 times, just until the butter-flour mixture is cut down to pea-sized pieces. Chill the dough in the freezer for 15 minutes.

3. Add the buttermilk to the food processor and mix well until it is just fully incorporated and the dough is moist and sticky. Scrape the dough into a bowl and press the dough into a ball. Cover the dough with plastic wrap and place in the refrigerator for 10 minutes.

4. Meanwhile, preheat the oven to 400°F.

5. Line a baking sheet with parchment paper. Drop biscuits, each about a ¼ cup in size, onto the prepared baking sheet. Bake for 15 to 17 minutes, until the biscuits are just starting to brown on top. Repeat with the remaining batter. Serve warm.

TIP

Keeping all the ingredients cold is the key to light and flaky biscuits. Also, if you don't want to cook them all at once you can keep the dough chilled in the fridge for up to 48 hours

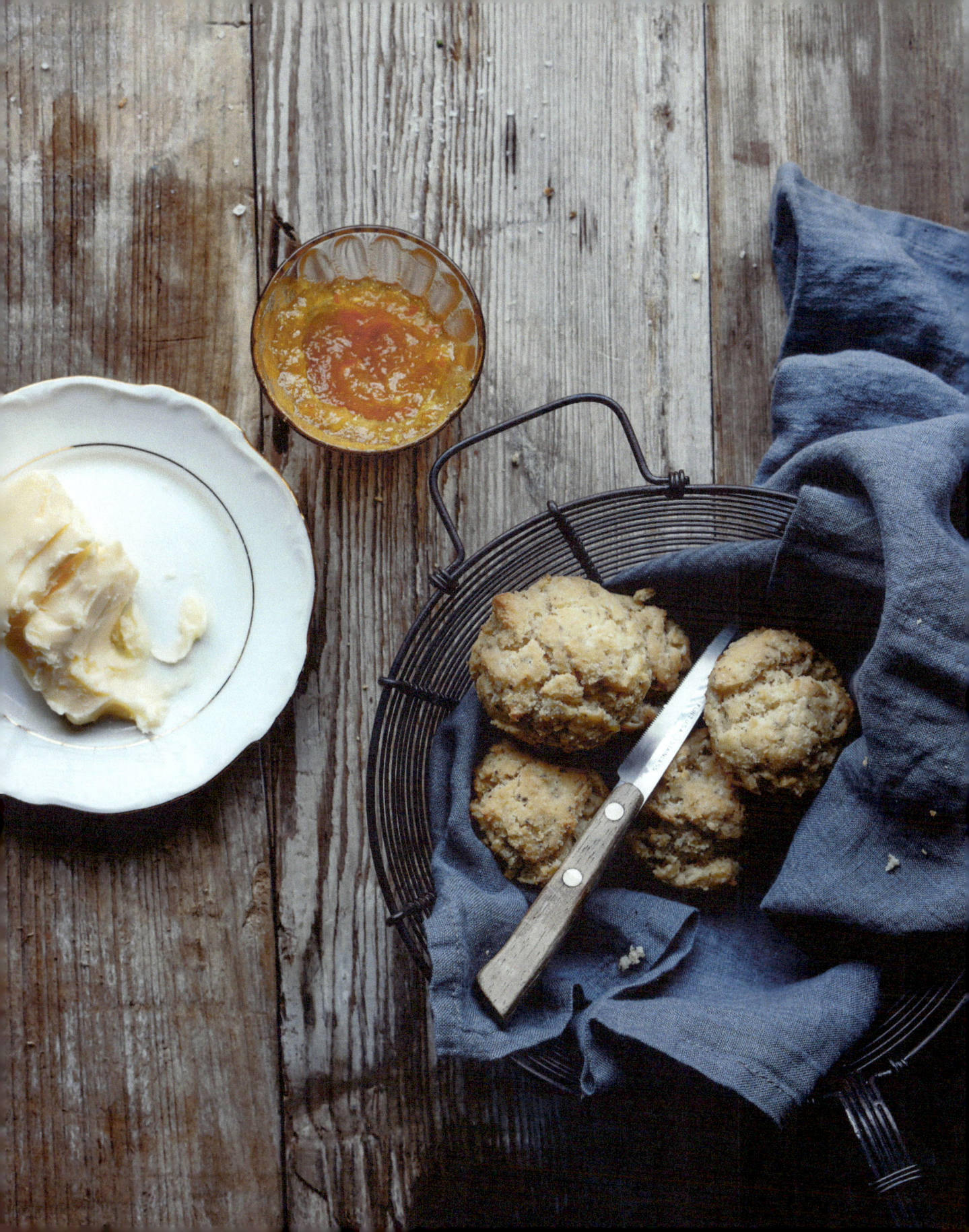

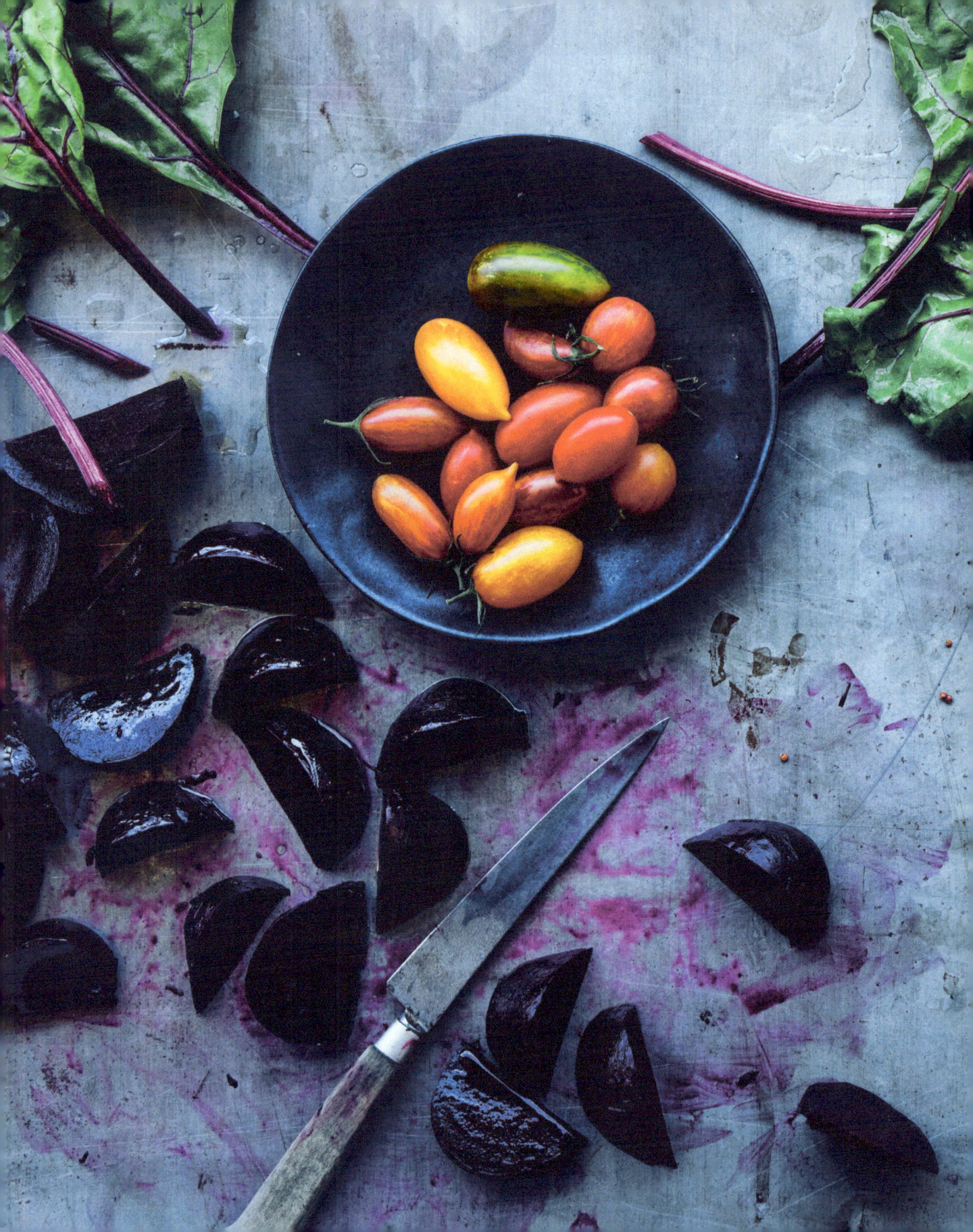

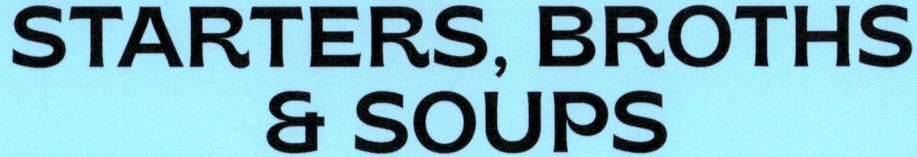

STARTERS, BROTHS & SOUPS

These recipes can be used as healthful meal starters or as hors d'oeuvres for entertaining. Our broths are a nutritional foundation to many dishes or gratifying on their own. We are also excited to share some of our most popular, easy-to-make soups that are great to kick off a meal or serve as a main event, especially to warm your bones during the colder months. Eat. Sip. Shine.

Move from the heart. Open it. Share its truth, its wisdom, its power. It is where we create from, heal from, grow from. Tap into it. It is infinite.

YAM BUTTER

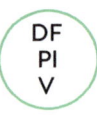

**DF
PI
V**

We could eat this all day long. It is a tasty substitute for regular butter for breads and crackers, a sandwich spread, a dipping sauce for veggies, or a garnish in soups. It is even a fantastic baby food!

Makes about 3 cups

4 yams (see Tip)
2 tablespoons extra-virgin olive oil
½ teaspoon sea salt

1. Preheat the oven to 400°F.

2. Scrub the yams until clean and dry them with a hand towel. Gently prick each yam with a fork several times.

3. Roast the yams in a baking dish for approximately 1 hour. The yams are done when you can easily pierce them with a fork. Let them cool for about 15 minutes.

4. Cut the yams in half and scoop out the flesh. Put into a food processor along with the olive oil and salt. Process until creamy, about 2 minutes. Store in an airtight container in the refrigerator for up to 5 days.

TIP

Make sure to use sweeter yams for a sweeter flavor.

CHEEZ SAUCE

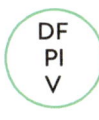

DF
PI
V

Makes about 2 cups

1½ cups raw cashew pieces
1 cup filtered water
¾ cup nutritional yeast
¼ teaspoon garlic powder
3 tablespoons fresh lemon juice
Sea salt to taste

1. Put the cashews in a bowl, cover with water, and soak for 6 hours orovernight. When the cashews are softened, rinse them thoroughly untilthe water runs clear.

2. Put the cashews in a food processor and process until smooth, approximately 2 minutes. Add the distilled water and continue to blend. Add the nutritional yeast, garlic powder, lemon juice, and sea salt and blend until all the ingredients are incorporated and the sauce is smooth. Store in an airtight container for up to 3 days

3. Serve over chopped fresh vegetables or radish chips (page 38).

TIP

If you do not have time to soak the cashews and are not concerned about the recipe being raw, put the cashews in a pot, cover with water, and simmer on low to medium heat for 15 to 20 minutes, until soft.

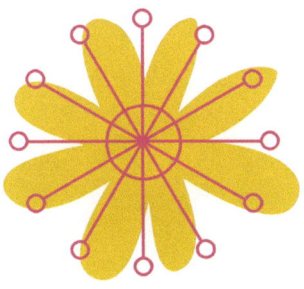

Jill: I feel like radishes are making a comeback, certainly in my kitchen but also in a world that's celebrating local produce and growing your own. They are blissfully easy to grow and mature quickly. Eating just-harvested radishes changed my perception of what once was for me a non-celebratory vegetable. Now I think of them as versatile, beautiful, tangy, sweet, juicy additions to any salad. I also love them prepared as an alternative to potato chips. The radish is back and ready for a party—serve them up with this arugula and sunflower pesto dipping sauce and you're sure to start one.

RADISH CHIPS WITH ARUGULA SUNFLOWER PESTO

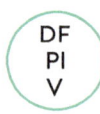

DF
PI
V

Serves 2 to 4

1 large bunch radishes, greens removed

2 tablespoons extra-virgin olive oil

Sea salt

Arugula Sunflower Pesto (p40)

1. Preheat the oven to 350°F.

2. Wash and dry the radishes thoroughly. Slice them with a mandoline or by hand. (Thinner slices will result in crunchier chips.) Toss with olive oil and salt.

3. Arrange the radish slices in a single layer on a baking sheet. Bake for 12 to 15 minutes, until crispy.

4. Let cool on the pan. Serve with the arugula pesto as a dipping sauce (see Tip p40).

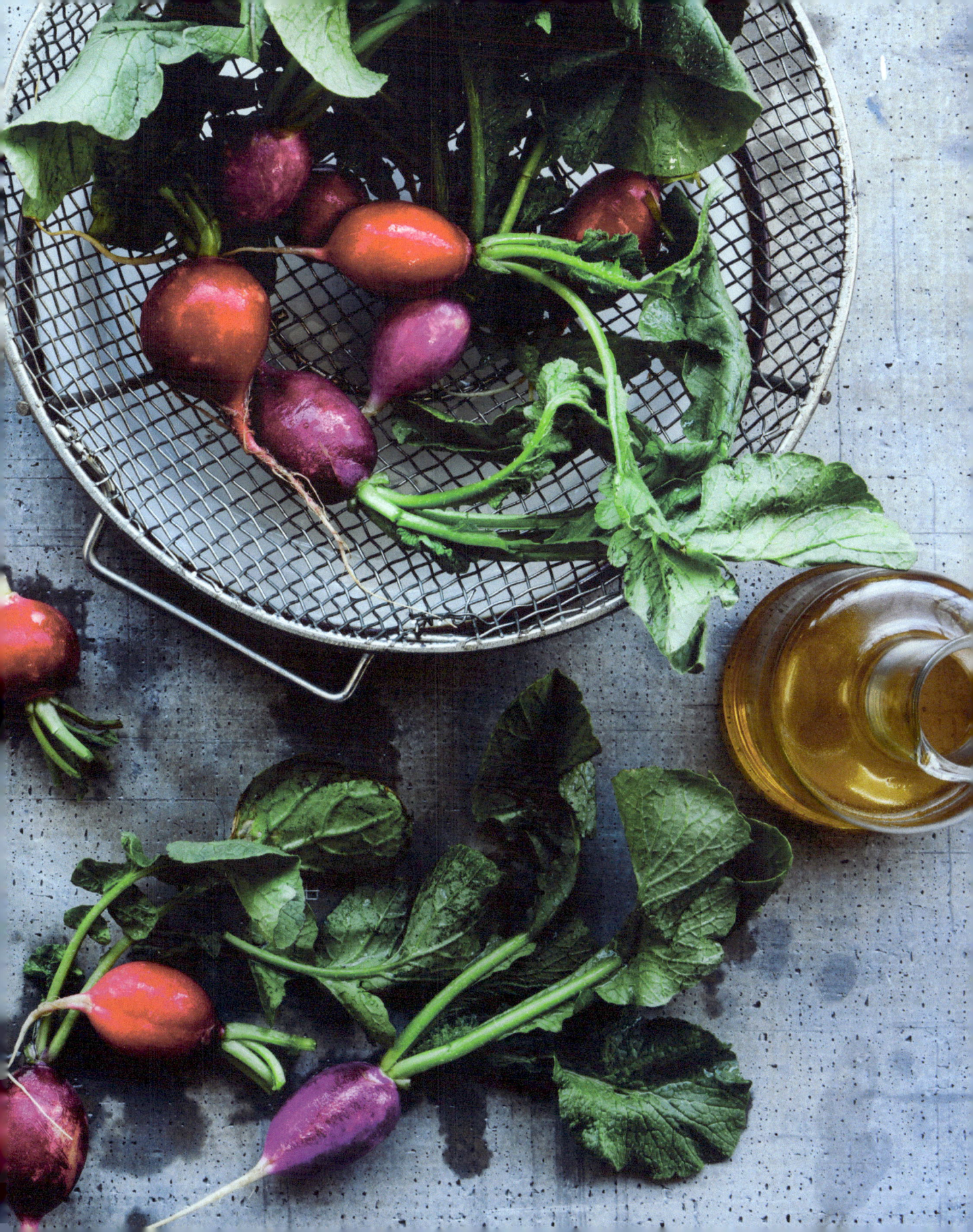

ARUGULA SUNFLOWER PESTO

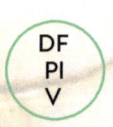

**DF
PI
V**

This is a fantastic dairy-free and nut-free alternative to regular pesto. The arugula adds a nice spiciness to sandwiches and pastas. We also enjoy it as a dip for our Radish Chips (p38) and even raw veggies. Nutritional yeast is a deactivated yeast that contains a wide spectrum of B vitamins and trace minerals. It works great in dairy-free dishes because it adds a "cheesy" flavor.

Makes about 2 cups

2 cloves garlic, peeled

¾ cup shelled sunflower seeds, soaked overnight then drained and rinsed

1 bunch arugula

Juice of 1 lemon

¼ cup nutritional yeast

½ cup extra-virgin olive oil

Sea salt to taste

1. Put the garlic and sunflower seeds in a food processor and process for 2 minutes. Add the arugula and lemon juice and process for 1 minute. Add the nutritional yeast and pulse until fully incorporated.

2. Slowly drizzle in the olive oil while processing until the pesto is smooth. Season with sea salt.

3. Serve immediately or store in a glass container. The pesto will keep in the refrigerator, covered tightly, for up to 5 days.

TIP

When the recipe is finished, check consistency to your liking. If you are looking for a thinner consistency, add 1 tablespoon of water at a time until you achieve your desired consistency.

WHY IS FERMENTATION ALL THE RAGE?

Fermentation, which can also be called culturing, is an age-old, tried-and-true method of preparing food that will help keep your body in optimal health. Some foods that we eat and drink regularly are certain breads, chocolate, and cheeses, certain teas, pickles, yogurt, sauerkrauts, kvass to name a few as well as wines, beer, and spirits (in moderation). The main reason we eat fermented food is to support digestion and promote a healthy gut, because this is the foundation of assimilation. Assimilation is how your body processes all of the nutrients that turn your food into fuel and that affects everything. Without good digestion, it doesn't matter what you eat, the cells just don't receive it.

Fermenting will help you assimilate your food. It's as simple as that, yet, we believe it is the key that unlocks the door to optimal health within your body and your life. Sandor Katz, who wrote the amazing book *The Art of Fermentation*, says "the creative space between fresh and rotten is the root of most of humanity's prized delicacies." It's true! Fermented food uses time and temperature to help good bacteria proliferate in foods, which not only helps preserve the food and deepen the flavors, but also helps heal our guts and keep our bodies balanced and healthy.

A simple way to think of it is that fermented foods are partially digested, which makes it very easy for our bodies to break them down and absorb their nutrients. Fermentation not only helps aid in digestion; it boosts the immune system, enhances the nutrient content of foods, and increases your body's energy to name a few of the benefits. And fermenting foods is surprisingly easy! In these days of processed foods and mass production, we have lost this ancient tradition and our bodies have suffered for it. Well now is the time to bring it back! Your belly is about to get really happy....

Raw cultured veggies are powerful superfoods. We've included quick and easy recipes for Cultured Salsa (page 46) and Cultured Carrots and Ginger (page 44). Adding just a quarter cup a day of these veggies to your diet will give you amazing health benefits, such as lowering the pH levels in your body to create a more alkaline environment. (Diseases thrive in acidic environments.) Always use clean organic vegetables for cultured recipes. If there are any pesticides or other chemicals in the vegetables, the toxins will become more concentrated during fermentation.

Soaking or sprouting your nuts, seeds, grains, and legumes is another form of fermentation; many examples of this are in the book. These techniques help release digestive enzymes, making even hard-to-digest foods much easier on our digestive systems so we can actually soak up all the nutrients these miracle foods have to offer. In fact, soaking and sprouting not only helps our bodies absorb vitamins, they actually increase the vitamin levels. Below are basic recipes for soaking nuts and sprouting seeds; no dehydrator or sprouting machine needed. If you choose, you can use soaked or sprouted ingredients even in recipes that don't specifically call for them.

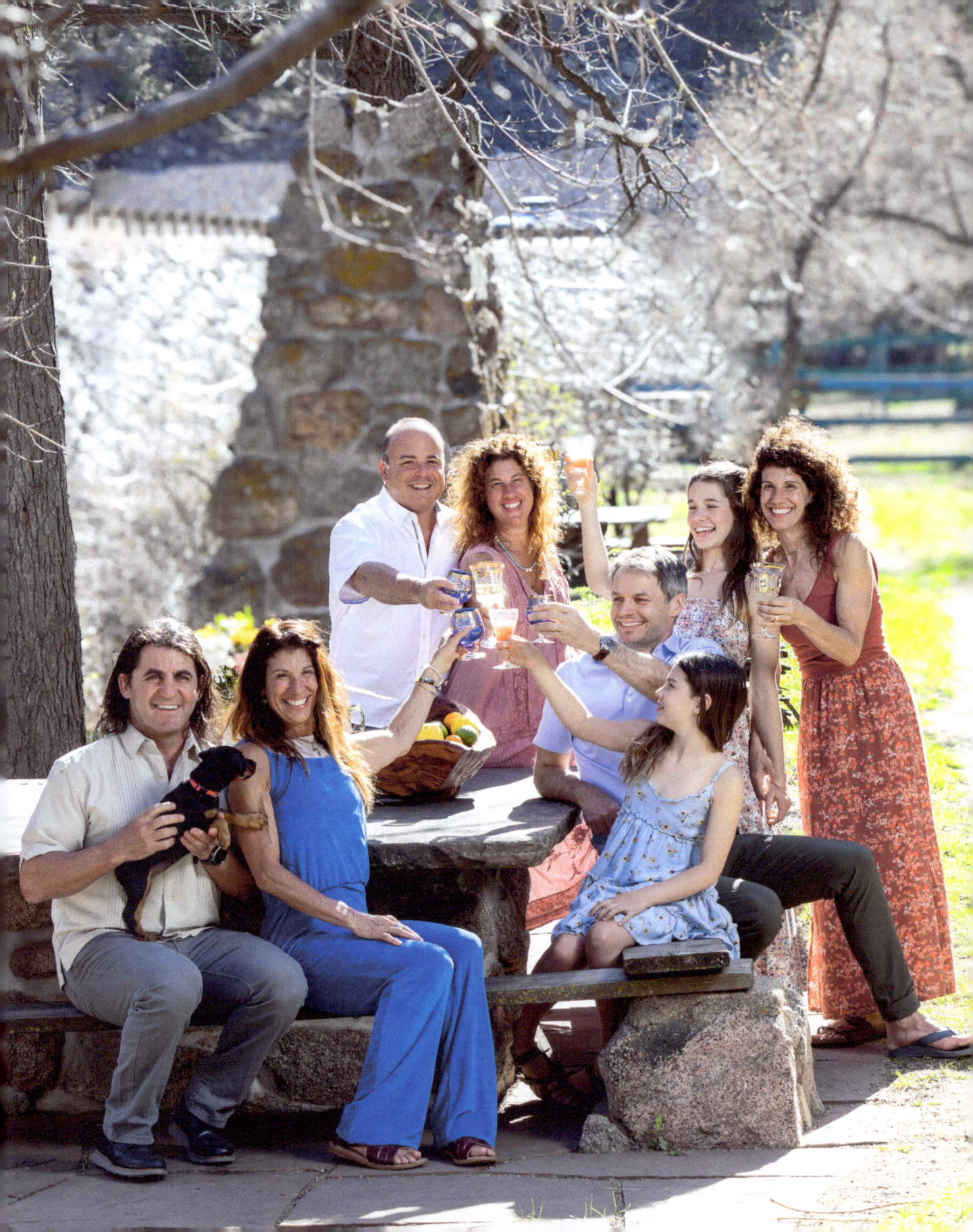

A BASIC RECIPE FOR SOAKING NUTS

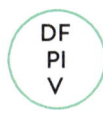

DF
PI
V

3 cups raw nuts, such as walnuts, almonds, or cashews

1 tablespoon sea salt

5 cups filtered water

2-quart mason ja

1. Combine the nuts and salt in a 2-quart mason jar and add the filtered water. Let the nuts soak for at least 7 hours or overnight.

2. Drain and rinse and lay out on a sheet pan.

3. Place the pan in a low-temperature oven (about 150°F). Let the nuts dry for approximately 7 hours, or until completely dry.

4. Store in the refrigerator in an airtight container. They will last approximately one month, depending on the type of nut.

A BASIC RECIPE FOR SPROUTING SEEDS

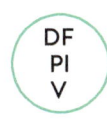

DF
PI
V

Makes about 1 cup

½ cup raw organic sprouting seeds, such as fenugreek, radish, or quinoa (see tip)

filtered water

2-quart mason jar with sprouting lid

1. Put the seeds in a mason jar and fill with enough water to cover the seeds. Put the sprouting lid on top and swirl the seeds and water to rinse the seeds and pour the water off while straining it through the lid.

2. Add more water using enough to cover the seeds by 4 inches and put the sprouting lid back on. Soak the seeds for at least 6 hours or overnight.

3. Rinse the seeds and drain well.

4. Let the seeds sit in the mason jar without water at room temperature for 24 to 72 hours to let them sprout. During this time, rinse the seeds every 6 to 8 hours. The sprouts are ready when you see a little tail that is approximately the same length as the original seed.

5. Rinse and drain the sprouts thoroughly and then store in the refrigerator for up to 5 days.

TIP

You need to use raw, whole, organic seeds for the sprouting process to be successful.

CULTURED CARROTS AND GINGER

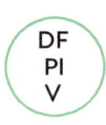
DF
PI
V

This is a sweet and tart garnish for seafood, salad, or soups. Just a tablespoon will aid in digestion. Culturing heightens the levels of nutrients that are already present in food, as well as adding enzymes and probiotics for gut health. See "Why Is Fermentation All the Rage?" on page 40 for more reasons why we are big fans of culturing.

*Makes one
64-ounce mason jar*

3 cups filtered water

3 tablespoons sea salt

2½ pounds fresh carrots, (about 20 medium), trimmed and cut into matchsticks or shredded

2 tablespoons peeled and minced fresh ginger

1 hefty outer cabbage leaf

1. To make the brine, bring 1 cup of the filtered water to a boil. Add the salt, stirring to dissolve. Once the salt is completely dissolved, add the remaining 2 cups of room temperature filtered water. Remove from the heat and let cool.

2. Combine the carrots and ginger in a sterilized half-gallon mason jar. Once the brine has cooled to room temperature, pour it over the carrot mixture, pushing the carrots down so that they are completely submerged in the brine.

3. Tightly and entirely cover the carrot and ginger mixture with the large cabbage leaf. This will help keep the fermentation process free of oxygen, which can cause mold. Leave 1 inch of headspace and screw on the lid.

4. Put the jar in a cool room or cupboard (65°F to 72°F is ideal). Allow the carrots to culture (ferment) for 7 to 10 days (see Tip), or as long as desired.

5. Refrigerate the jar after opening. The cultured carrots will last for up to 3 months in the refrigerator.

TIP

Make sure to "burp" your jar every day for the first 3 or 4 days of the fermentation process to let the gas escape. Do this by unscrewing the cap, removing it for a couple of seconds, and then screwing on the cap securely again. Sterilize your jar either in your dishwasher or by boiling the jars in a large pot.

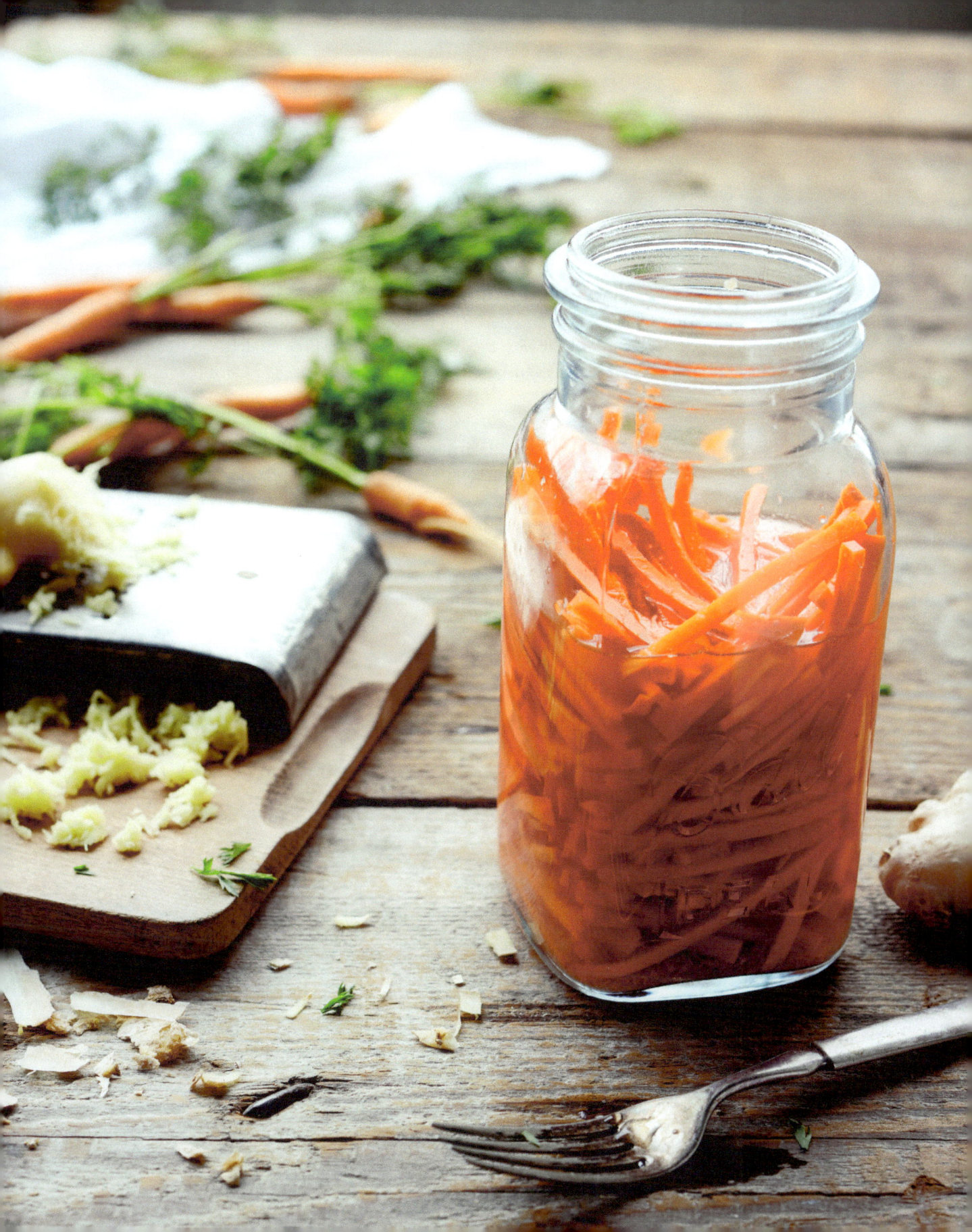

CULTURED SALSA

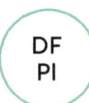

DF
PI

Everyone loves chips and salsa, and we have mastered a way to up the ante on digestion and the health benefits of the tomatoes through fermentation. The longer this salsa cultures, the more flavor it has. Serve it with tacos, chips, or Bean-Free Chili (page 106), Avocado Mash (page 23), Baked Eggs in Avocado Cups (page 22), or fish dishes.

Makes about 6 cups

3 pounds ripe tomatoes, cut into medium dice (About 6 cups—we love roma tomatoes for this recipe)

1 small onion, diced

2 tablespoons chopped cilantro

2½ tablespoons sliced green onions

1½ tablespoons minced garlic

1 tablespoon seeded and minced jalapeño

1 teaspoon ground cumin, toasted briefly in a skillet just until fragrant

¼ cup fresh lime juice

1 tablespoon sea salt

Put all the ingredients in a large bowl and stir to combine. Pour into a clean half-gallon mason jar and screw on the lid. Put the jar in a cool spot, ideally between 65°F and 72°F, for 2 to 3 days, depending on your preference in flavor. As it sits longer, the flavor becomes brighter and more effervescent. After culturing, store in a glass container and refrigerate for up to 10 days.

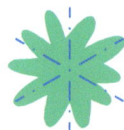

TIP

Topping with a cabbage leaf as in the Cultured Carrots and Ginger is not necessary for this ferment. The acid in the tomatoes and lime help protect from mold, and the shorter fermentation time also reduces the possibility of mold. You can also skip the fermentation process for a simple delicious salsa that you can eat right away!

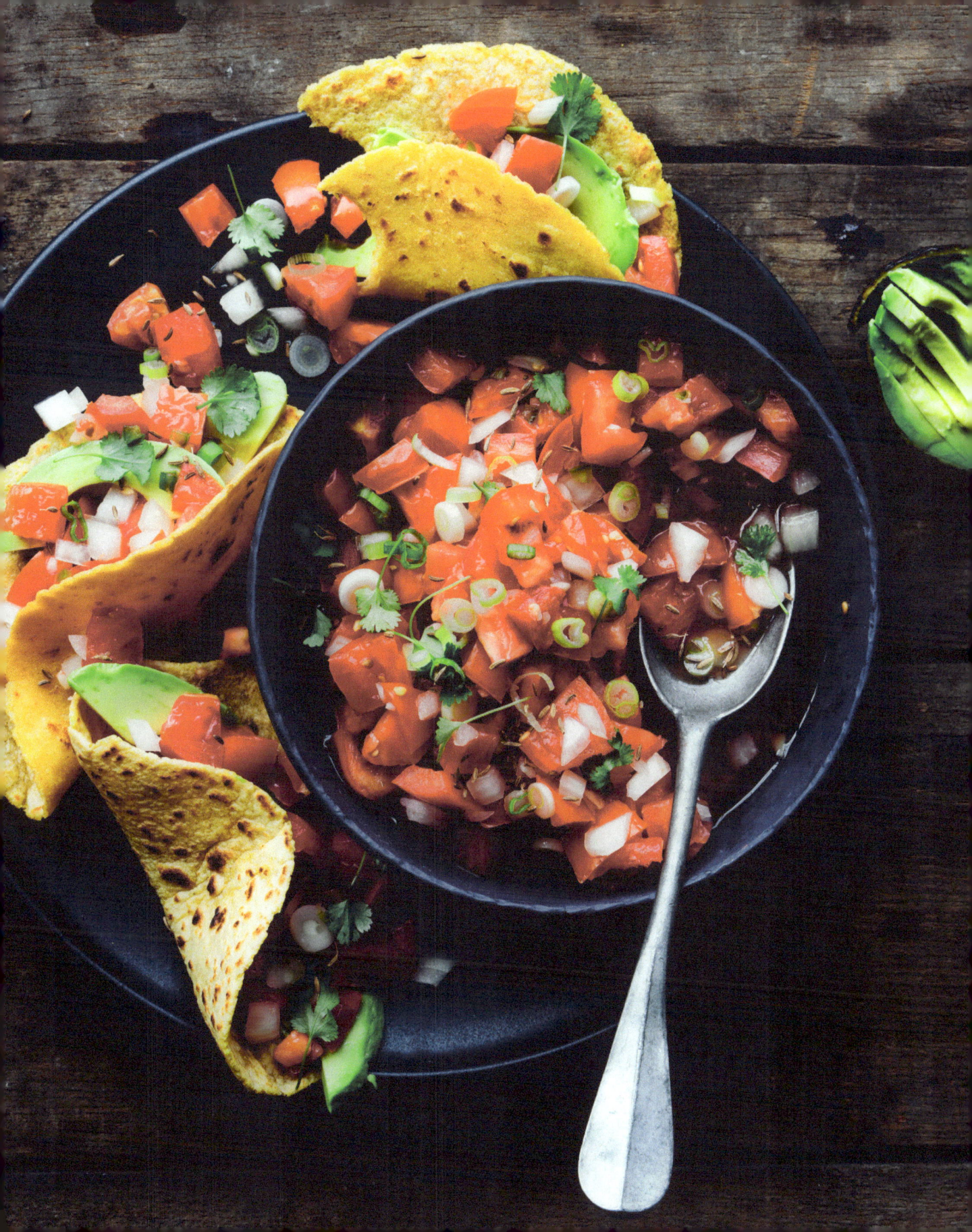

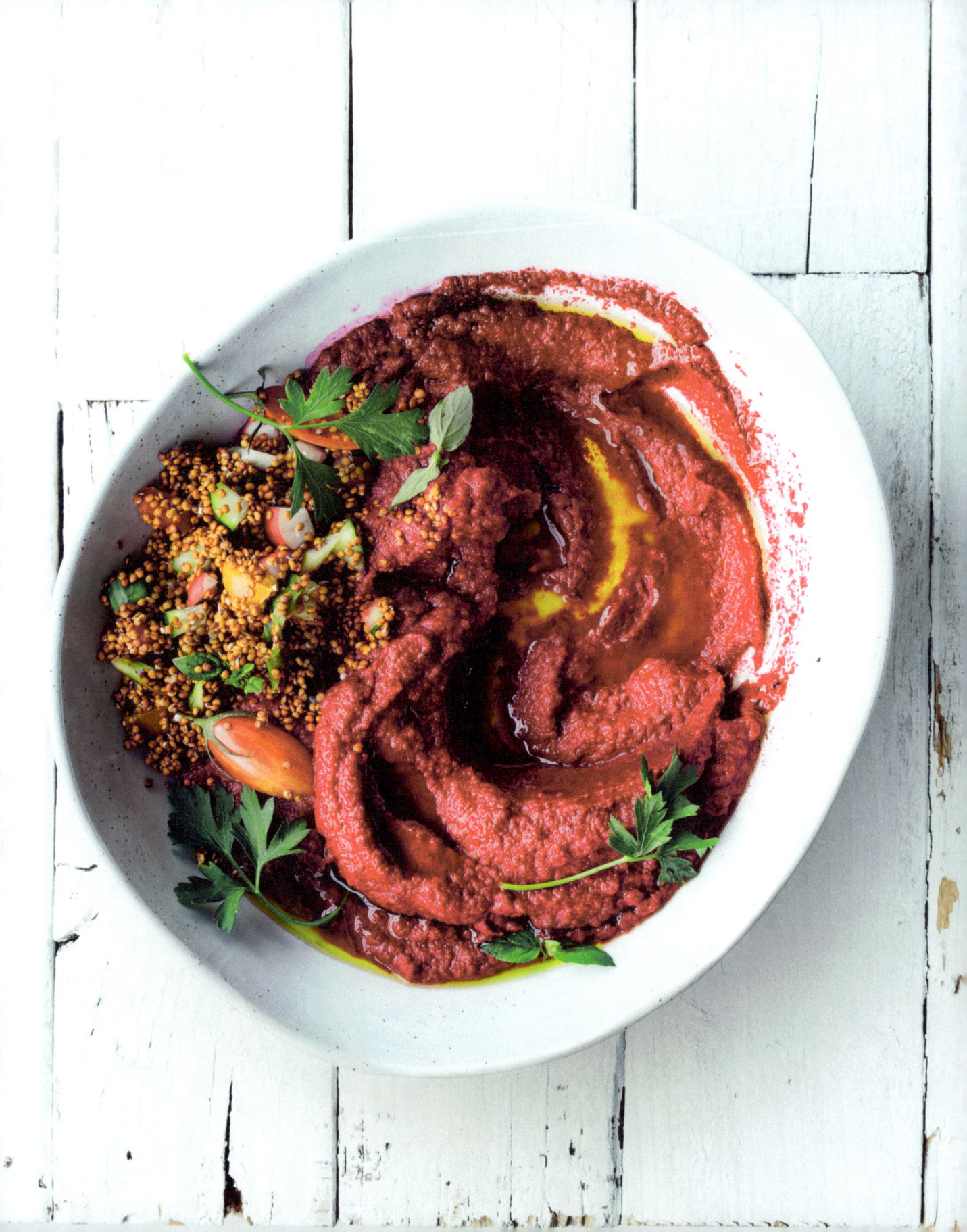

BEET HUMMUS

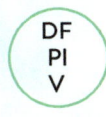

DF
PI
V

Makes about 2½ cups

4 medium beets,
peels on, scrubbed
to remove any dirt

2 tablespoons extra-
virgin olive oil

½ cup water

Sea salt to taste

¼ cup tahini (sesame
seed paste)

¼ cup fresh lemon juice

1 to 2 cloves garlic,
coarsely chopped
(see Tip)

1. Preheat the oven to 375°F.

2. Rub the whole beets with olive oil and a touch of salt. Put them on a baking pan, pour in the water and roast covered with foil for approximately 1 hour, until the beets are easily pierced through with a fork. Let cool slightly.

3. When the beets are cool enough to handle, rub the skins off with a clean dishcloth (be forewarned—the beets will stain it) or use a vegetable peeler. Coarsely chop the beets and put in them food processor with the remaining ingredients. Blend until smooth.

4. Serve with your favorite chopped veggies or flatbread. Refrigerate leftovers, if any, in an airtight container for up to 5 days.

TIP

Since the garlic is raw, it will add a pungent garlic flavor to the hummus. You can use just 1 clove, if you prefer, or roast the garlic for a softer flavor.

Jennifer: Beets have always been a favorite of mine. I love their deep color. This hummus was eye candy on the table at our restaurants, where it was one of our most popular shared appetizers. It has no beans—just the beauty of the beets, sesame seed paste, garlic, and lemon.

RAW SPROUTED QUINOA TABOULI

Because this tabouli is completely raw, yet sprouted, it is a highly digestible and power-packed superfood! Sprouted seeds are rich in enzymes, which are healing for the body and also help digest everything you eat with them. Quinoa is technically a seed, which makes it higher in protein than grains. We serve this recipe at our restaurant with our beet hummus; it is also great on sandwiches, salads, and fish. The herbs and crunch from the radishes, cucumber, and tomatoes add a vibrant texture to the tabouli.

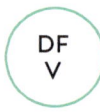

Makes about 4 cups

1 cup dry quinoa, soaked overnight in water until sprouted (about 12 hours; see Tip)

¼ cup radishes, diced

¼ cup cucumber, diced

¼ cup cherry tomatoes, diced

¼ cup scallions, cut on a diagonal into small pieces

¼ cup chopped fresh parsley

¼ cup chopped fresh mint

1 clove garlic, minced

¼ cup fresh lemon juice

½ cup extra-virgin olive oil

Sea salt to taste

1. Drain and rinse the quinoa then put it in a mixing bowl. Add the radishes, cucumber, tomatoes, scallions, parsley, and mint and toss to combine.

2. In a small bowl, whisk together the garlic, lemon juice, and olive oil. Pour the dressing over the quinoa mixture and toss to coat. Season with salt.

3. Leftovers may be stored in the fridge for up to 4 days.

TIP

If the temperature of your kitchen is too cool, the quinoa sometimes doesn't sprout in the 12 hours specified in the recipe. If you do not see a small sprout coming from the seed, drain and rinse the quinoa anyway, but put the seeds back in your soaking container without water and let them sit in the container for another 6 to 8 hours or overnight. They should be sprouted by then. Rinse and continue with the recipe. If you prefer, you can also cook and cool the quinoa rather than sprout it and make the same recipe with the cooked quinoa.

KALE CHIPS

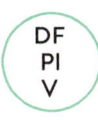

DF
PI
V

These kale chips are crunchy, tender, savory, and addictive—an easy way to get kids and adults eating one of the most nutrient-dense foods on the planet. They are great with sandwiches as an alternative to potato chips. They also do well as a side to steak, chicken, or fish.

Serves 2 to 4

1 bunch kale (lacinato, dinosaur, or Tuscan)

1 tablespoon coconut oil

½ tablespoon gluten-free tamari

1½ tablespoons nutritional yeast

1. Preheat the oven to 375°F.

2. Wash the kale leaves and dry them well. (You can use a salad spinner and then blot the leaves dry on a kitchen towel.) To destem the kale, hold a piece of kale by the stem in one hand, then starting at the stem end, run your other hand along the length, ripping off the leaves off as you go (see Tip). Repeat with the rest of the kale. Cut or tear the leaves into bite-size pieces and put them in a bowl.

3. Add the coconut oil and tamari to the kale and massage for 2 minutes, until the kale is soft and slightly darker.

4. Spread the kale out on 2 ungreased baking sheets, put both in the oven, and set the timer for 4 minutes. Pull the kale out of the oven and sprinkle with the nutritional yeast, give it a quick mix, and put it back in the oven for 4 minutes more until crispy.

5. Transfer the kale chips to a platter and serve immediately. Or let them cool thoroughly, then store them in a tightly covered mason jar or glass container. They'll stay crispy for up to 3 days.

TIP

The kale stems can be saved and used in smoothies or in Pressed Green Juice (page 149). For an Italian-style version, flavor the kale leaves with garlic salt, Romano cheese (if you eat dairy), and lemon juice before baking..

THE BEEF ON BROTHS: BONE AND VEGETABLE BROTHS

Bone broths and vegetable broths are amazing elixirs that provide vitamins and minerals that are easily absorbed into our bodies. The inner part of the bones contains astounding health benefits, and slow-cooking them in water releases all of their goodness into the broth. Vegetables that are cooked in this way also release a rich nutritional content, too, and they are very alkalizing, which helps keeps your body in a healthy balance. Broths and stocks can be used as a base for soups and sauces or sipped throughout the day like a tea. Vegetable broth can be can be seasoned with sea salt before sipping.

Bone broths are high in gelatin, which is beneficial to our hair, skin, nails, joints, connective tissue, and also our guts. They help heal our intestines and are especially beneficial to those dealing with leaky gut and other digestive ailments. They are high in trace minerals that may be hard to get from other sources. For those people that don't eat dairy, they provide a solid dose of calcium. When regularly drinking vegetable and bone broths, you will notice clearer skin, your digestion will be on track, and it will absolutely help with inflammation or pain in the body. It also helps curb hunger. They are amazing for an all-around healthy immune system and deeply healing for the body.

You can start with either raw bones or cooked (meaning if you roast a whole chicken, you can repurpose the bones to make a broth). For vegetables, start with organic raw vegetables. Using bones from organic grass-fed cattle, sheep, and free-range chickens and using organic vegetables is important here. You are slow-cooking to pull out all of the components of the ingredients, so you want to make sure they are clean and pure with no added chemicals, hormones, or antibiotics. Using apple cider vinegar during the cooking process of bone broths helps to draw the minerals out of the bones to get the optimal amount of nutrients from them.

Broths and stocks are some of the most nourishing foods you can put in your body. They hydrate, heal, and load you up with tons and tons of minerals, warding off colds and sickness. For optimal health and all-around wellness, why not make broths a part of your everyday routine? Your body will thank you!

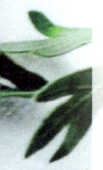
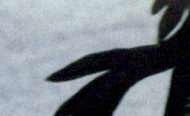

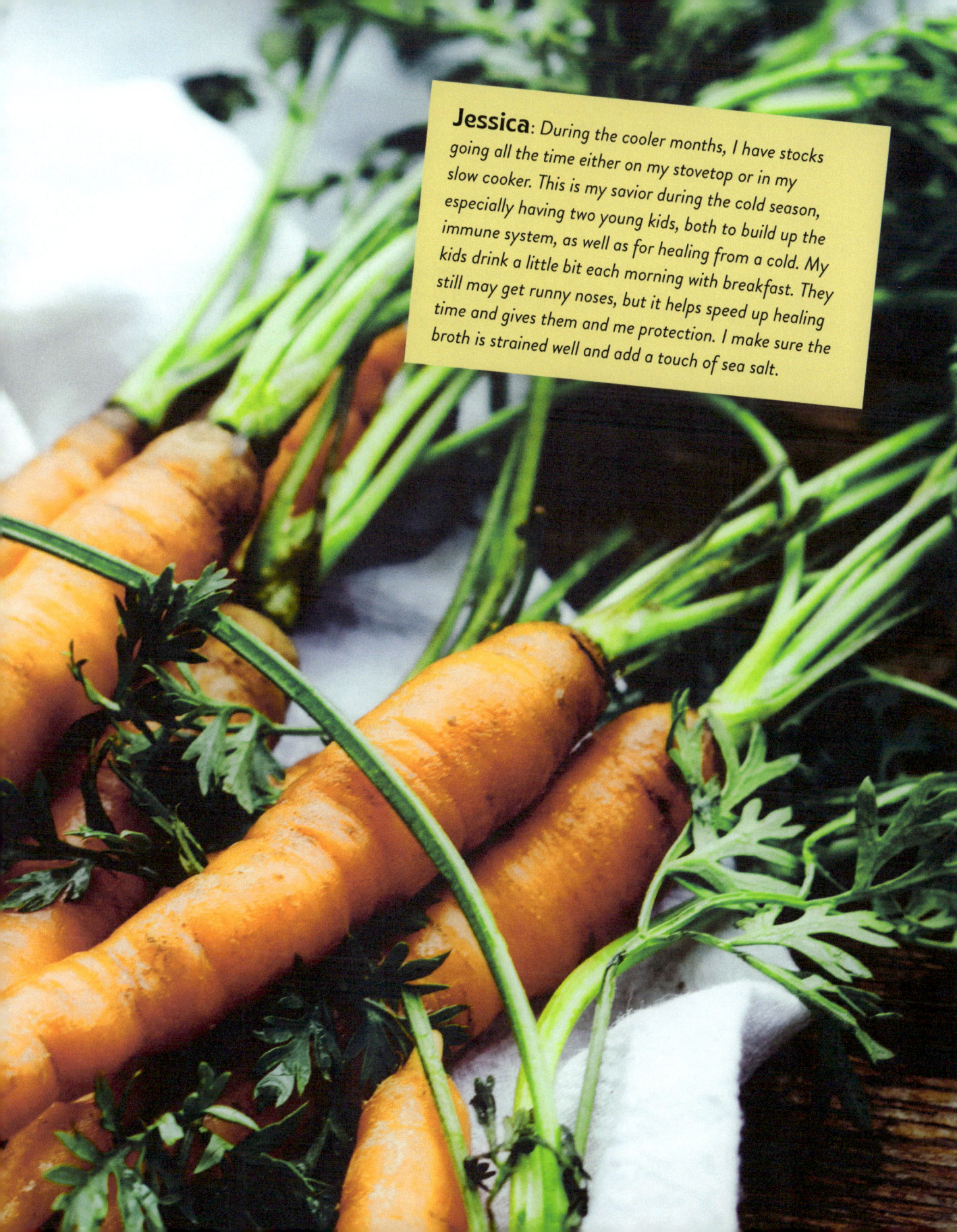

Jessica: During the cooler months, I have stocks going all the time either on my stovetop or in my slow cooker. This is my savior during the cold season, especially having two young kids, both to build up the immune system, as well as for healing from a cold. My kids drink a little bit each morning with breakfast. They still may get runny noses, but it helps speed up healing time and gives them and me protection. I make sure the broth is strained well and add a touch of sea salt.

VEGETABLE BROTH

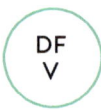

**DF
V**

Vegetable broth can be seasoned with sea salt and sipped throughout the day or used as a base for soups and sauces. We like the addition of seaweed to add to the mineral content and flavor of this broth.

*Makes about
2 quarts*

1 small onion, chopped

2 medium carrots, chopped

3 stalks celery, chopped

2 large cloves garlic, crushed

½ bunch kale or Swiss chard (chard will turn your broth a light purple)

½ cup mushroom stems

1 handful fresh flat-leaf parsley leaves

1 large piece seaweed, preferably dulse or wakame, (optional)

about 10 cups filtered water, or more if needed to cover ingredients

1. Combine all of the ingredients in a large stockpot, making sure there is enough water to cover the vegetables completely, and bring to a boil. Lower the heat and simmer for 1½ to 2 hours (see Tip). Remove from the heat and let cool for about 20 minutes so it is easier to handle.

2. Strain the stock through a fine-mesh sieve into one or several airtight containers. Refrigerate for up to 5 days, or freeze for future use.

TIP

We like using tempered mason jars to store stock. They can handle the heat. If you are freezing the stock, leave at least 3 inches at the top of the jar to allow room for expansion. Vegetable broths are simmered for a shorter amount of time than bone broths because they can get bitter if cooked too long. Also, when cooking bones, you need a longer amount of cooking time to draw out the minerals and flavor. This happens much more quickly with vegetable broths.

BEEF BONE BROTH

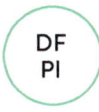

DF
PI

We always use organic bones from grass-fed animals when we make our beef bone broth. Beef broth is richer, darker, and meatier than chicken broth, so keep that in mind as you use it in soups and other recipes.

Makes about 2 quarts

1 tablespoon extra-virgin olive oil

2 pounds grass-fed beef bones with marrow

¾ cup tomato paste (see Tip)

2 tablespoons raw apple cider vinegar

about 10 cups filtered water, or more if needed to cover ingredients

1 medium onion, coarsely chopped

2 small carrots, peeled and coarsely chopped

2 stalks celery, coarsely chopped

5 sprigs parsley

5 sprigs thyme

1 bay leaf

1. Preheat the oven to 400°F.

2. Lightly grease a baking pan with the olive oil. Spread the bones out on the pan and brush them liberally with the tomato paste. Roast the bones for about 25 minutes, turning them once so they brown on all sides.

3. In a large stockpot, combine the roasted bones, vinegar, and distilled water, making sure there is enough water to cover the bones. Bring to a boil. Lower the heat and simmer for 4 to 6 hours, occasionally skimming off any foam that comes to the top and adding more water if needed to keep bones covered.

4. Add the onion, carrots, celery, parsley, thyme, and bay leaf and continue to cook for another 2 hours. Remove from the heat and let cool for about 20 minutes for easier handling.

5. Strain the stock through a fine-mesh sieve into one or several airtight containers and put them in the refrigerator to chill.

6. Skim off the fat that congeals on the top as it chills. Refrigerate the stock for up to 5 days, or freeze for future use.

TIP

If you have a sensitivity to nightshades, you may leave the tomato paste out, as it is mainly included to add sweetness to the broth..

CHICKEN BONE BROTH

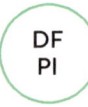

DF
PI

Ask your butcher for high-quality organic and free-range chicken bones (or you can even use the bones from roasted chicken). Broths are great to keep your immune system strong and to help heal a common cold and body inflammation. We enjoy this chicken broth as a sipping tea or as a base for sauces or soups. See "The Beef on Broths" (page 52) for more information about the uses and powerful benefits of broths.

*Makes about
2 quarts*

2 pounds bony chicken parts (bone-in necks, backs, wings, and thighs)

gizzards of 1 chicken (optional)

1 tablespoon raw apple cider vinegar

about 10 cups filtered water, or more if needed to cover ingredients

1 medium onion, coarsely chopped

2 small carrots, peeled and coarsely chopped

2 stalks celery, coarsely chopped

5 sprigs parsley

5 sprigs thyme

1 bay leaf

1. In a large stockpot, combine the bones, gizzards, if using, vinegar, and distilled water, making sure there is enough water to cover the bones. Bring to a boil. Lower the heat and simmer for 4 to 6 hours (see Tip), occasionally skimming off any foam that comes to the surface and adding more water if needed to keep bones covered.

2. Add the onion, carrots, celery, parsley, thyme, and bay leaf and continue to simmer for another 2 hours. Remove from the heat and let cool for about 20 minutes so that it is easier to handle.

3. Strain the stock through a fine-mesh sieve into one or several airtight containers and put them in the refrigerator to chill.

4. Skim off the fat that congeals on the top as it cools. Refrigerate the stock for up to 5 days, or freeze for future use.

TIP

The longer you cook the chicken bones, the richer and more flavorful the stock will be. However, it is best to cook the vegetables for a maximum of 2 hours.

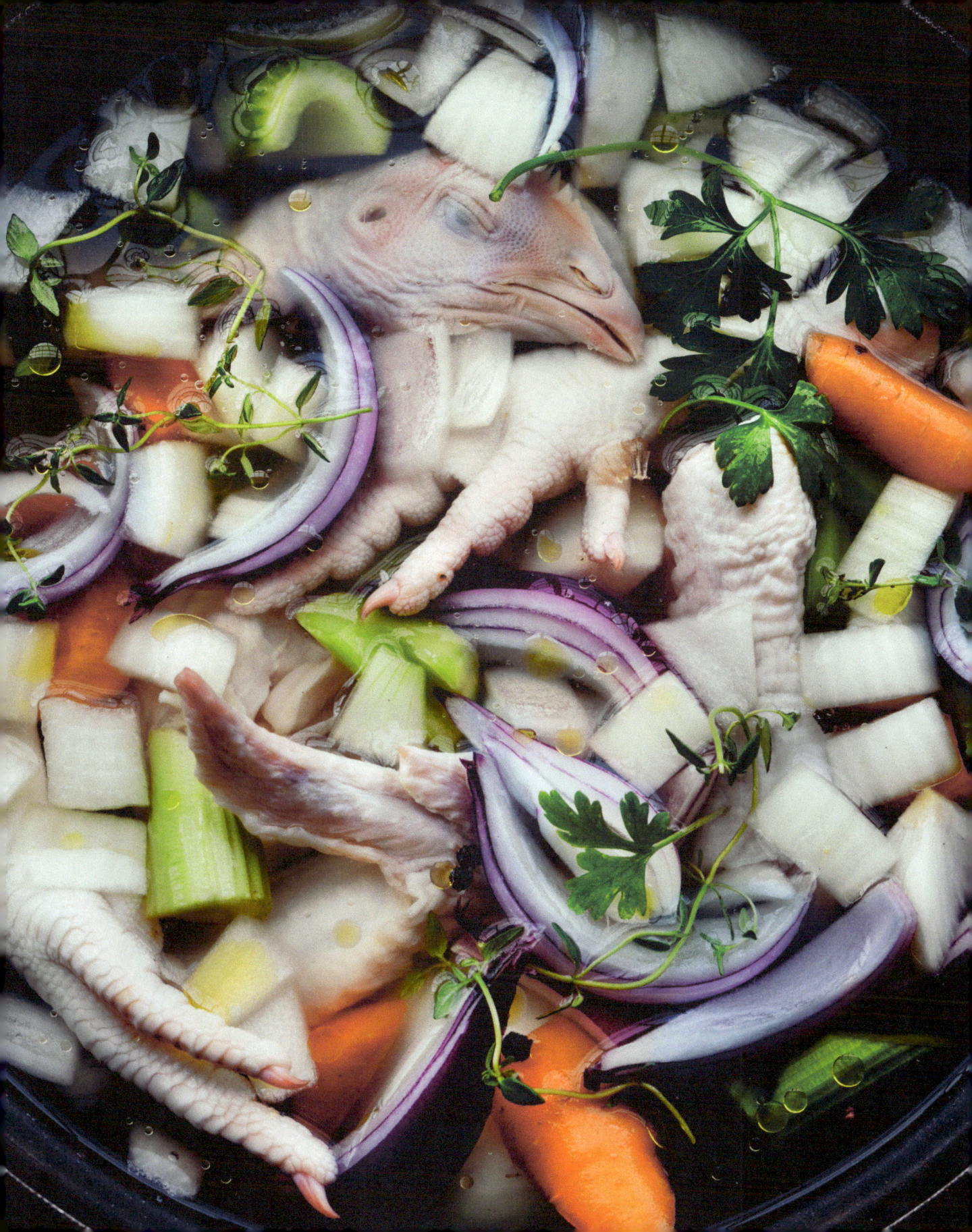

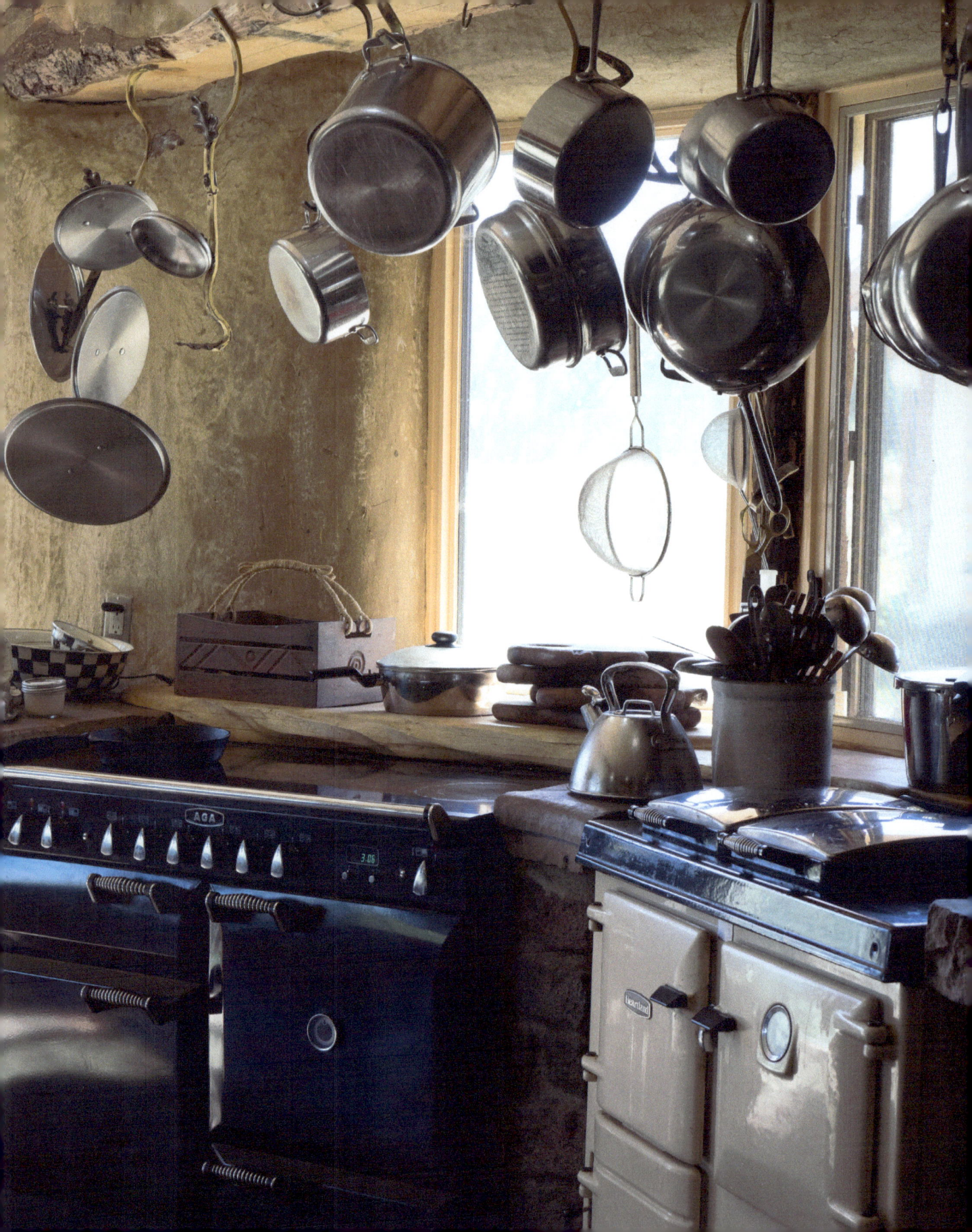

SQUASH AND PEAR SOUP WITH SPICED COCONUT MILK

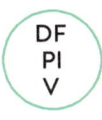

DF
PI
V

This is a fall soup that nourishes the lungs and warms the body. It is the perfect soup to serve at the start of the cooler weather, when we are more susceptible to colds. This soup hits the right balance between spiced and sweet that is pleasing to every generation. Plus, it just feels good going down.

Serves 6 to 8

1 (3-pound) acorn or butternut squash

2 tablespoons coconut oil, plus more for brushing

¼ cup chopped yellow onion

1 stalk celery, chopped

2 pears, peeled, seeded, and chopped

sea salt to taste

4 cups vegetable or chicken stock (to make your own, see page 54 or 56)

½ cup full-fat canned coconut milk

¼ cup maple syrup

1 teaspoon peeled and minced fresh ginger

1 teaspoon ground cinnamon

1 pinch ground nutmeg

2 teaspoons vanilla extract (to make your own, see page 163)

3 tablespoons chopped raw pecans

1. Preheat the oven to 350°F.

2. Cut the squash in half lengthwise and scoop out the seeds. Brush the fleshy sides with coconut oil and place, flesh down, on a baking sheet. Bake until tender, 35 to 40 minutes.

3. Meanwhile, heat the coconut oil in a soup pot and sauté the onion, celery, and pear with a bit of salt until softened and lightly caramelized.

4. Add the stock to the pot and simmer for 30 minutes, uncovered.

5. Scoop the roasted squash out of the peel and add to the simmering stock. Stir in the coconut milk, maple syrup, ginger, cinnamon, nutmeg, and vanilla and simmer for another 30 minutes.

6. Puree the soup with a high-powered hand blender or in batches in a high-powered blender until smooth. Start blending slowly first before running at a higher speed to avoid splashing hot soup.

7. Serve in bowls garnished with the pecans.

TIP

For a hearty main dish, add some protein to this soup by including a scoop of pulled chicken or beef in the center of each bowl.

VEGAN WILD MUSHROOM BISQUE

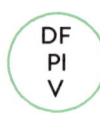

DF
PI
V

Serves 6 to 8

1 small head cauliflower, florets separated and chopped

5 tablespoons extra-virgin olive oil

sea salt to taste

1½ cups raw cashew pieces, rinsed (see Tip)

1 large apple, chopped

2 cups chopped assorted mushrooms.

1 shallot, minced

½ cup white wine

1 teaspoon fresh thyme leaves

2 teaspoons minced fresh sage

6 cups vegetable stock (to make your own, see page 54)

1 pinch ground nutmeg

1. Preheat the oven to 375°F.

2. In a mixing bowl, toss the cauliflower with 3 tablespoons of the olive oil and season with salt. Pour onto a baking sheet and roast until tender and lightly browned, approximately 20 minutes.

3. Rinse the cashews, place in a small pot, and add enough water to cover. Bring the cashews to a boil and then lower the heat and simmer for 30 minutes.

4. Meanwhile, heat the remaining 2 tablespoons olive oil in a wide-bottomed pot. Add the apples and mushrooms with a dash of salt and sauté until soft and caramelized. Add the shallot and sauté for another 5 minutes. Pour the wine into the pot and simmer until the liquid is reduced by two-thirds.

5. Stir in the roasted cauliflower, thyme, and sage. Add the vegetable stock (see Tip) and bring to a boil. Lower the heat and simmer for 30 minutes.

6. Meanwhile, drain and rinse the cooked cashews. Put the cashews in a highpowered blender and add just enough water to cover them. Blend on high speed until the cashew mixture is silky smooth and creamy. Pulse in the nutmeg.

7. Working in batches, puree the soup with the cashew cream in a blender or with a hand blender until smooth. Return the soup to the pot and simmer for 10 minutes more to develop the flavors.

TIP

We like to rinse nuts and seeds before using them to remove any debris or residue. You can play with the consistency of the bisque by adding or reducing the amount of veggie stock you add.

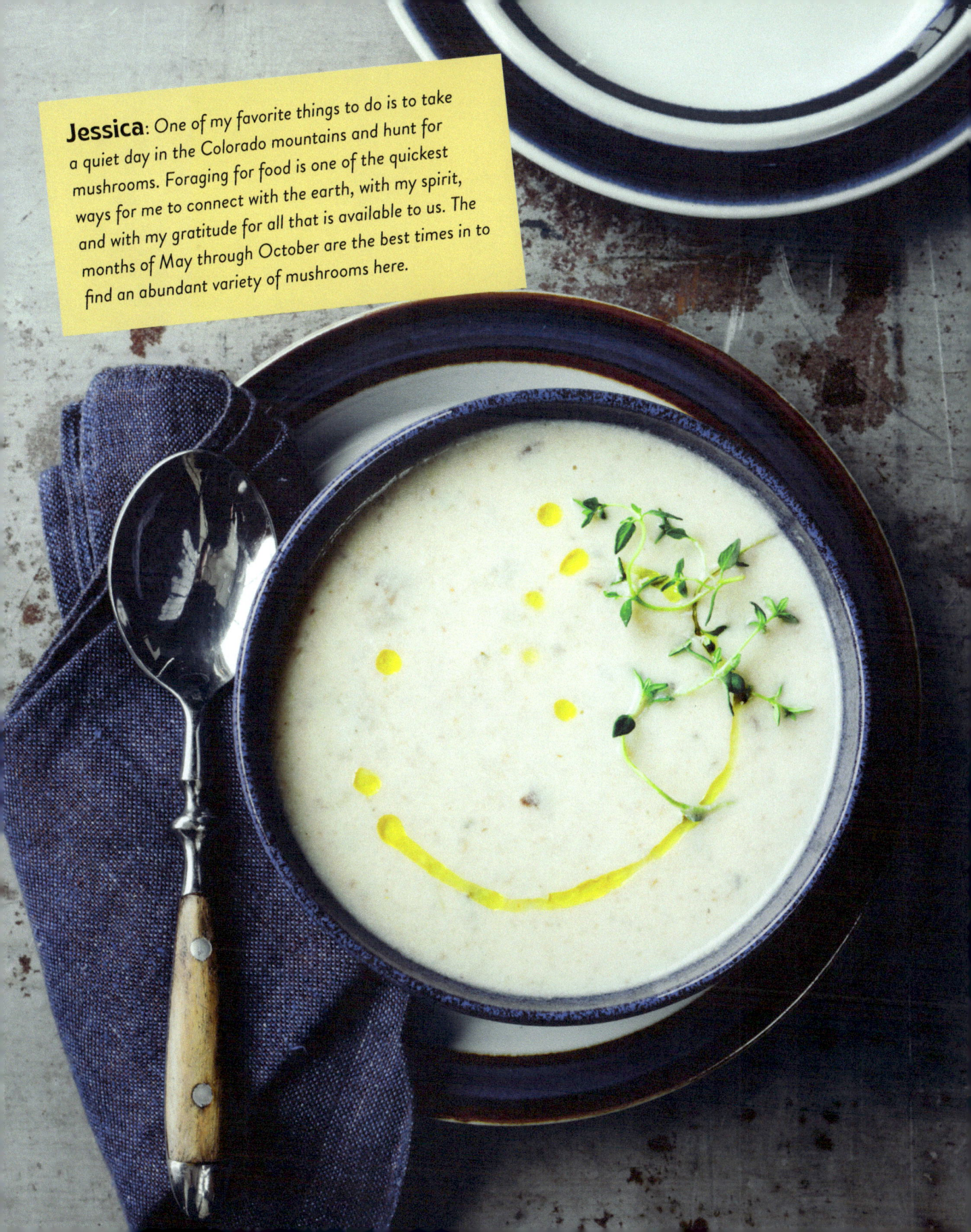

Jessica: One of my favorite things to do is to take a quiet day in the Colorado mountains and hunt for mushrooms. Foraging for food is one of the quickest ways for me to connect with the earth, with my spirit, and with my gratitude for all that is available to us. The months of May through October are the best times in to find an abundant variety of mushrooms here.

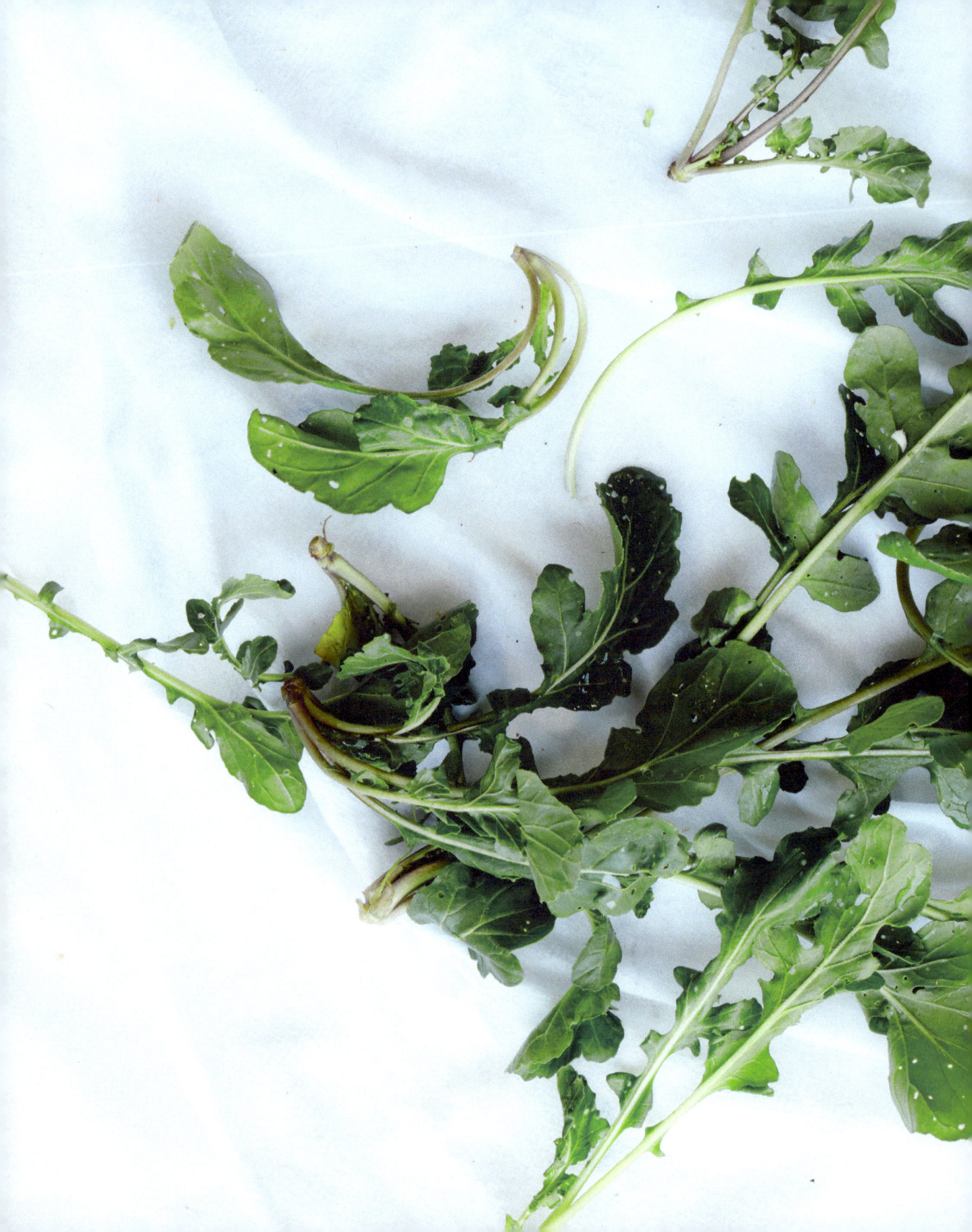

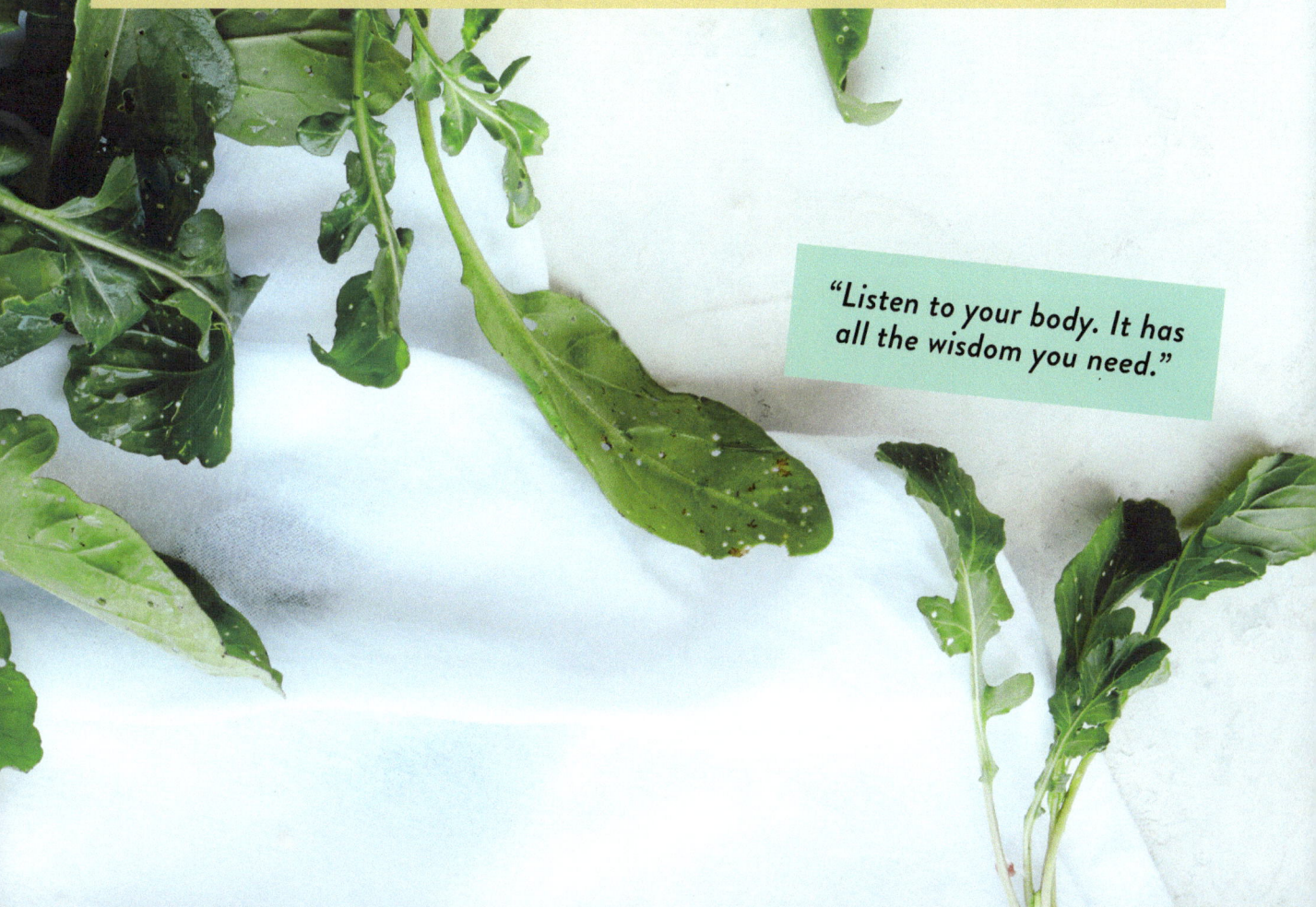

ALL DRESSED UP

We have an ongoing love affair with creative salads. This is where seasonality and local ingredients get really fun. Eating with the seasons is something we are very passionate about. As a matter of fact, we have built our restaurants around this concept. Eating what is in season is the most nutritious way of eating because eating seasonally typically leads to eating locally. And when you can buy food more locally, not only does it have more nutritional value, but it also tastes better. There is nothing like eating an apple that has been picked fresh off a tree rather than one that has been flown across the world. Eating locally also supports your local economy and helps connects you to your food and where it is coming from.

"Listen to your body. It has all the wisdom you need."

WHY WE DIG ON WHOLE FOODS

When the three of us went off to college, it was at the height of the low-fat, low-carb craze that seemed to have swept the nation. The truth of the matter is, each of us was at the heaviest weight we have ever been. In our fridges and cupboards, there was everything from low-fat sour cream and fat-free chips to low-fat cheeses—if it came in low fat, we were on it. Hip-hip-hooray, a shortcut to keeping all things "light!" The more we indulged, the more the pounds packed on. It took some time to come to grips with it, to put down the "lite" beer and the bag of fat-free potato chips and ask, "Ok, what gives?" This was a shortcut that was not working.

Right around that time, we took a family trip along Highway 1 through California. Individually we were each having an eye-opening experience: Looking at all the farms as they passed by and taking in the artichokes and cabbages, herds of cows and stands with tons of veggies, meats, raw milk, and yogurts, we thought how vibrant and beautiful the food looked and how ALIVE. It got us talking about organic foods, local foods, and whole foods. It got us thinking about the effect of what we put in our mouths and bodies. The food at these farms was beautiful and tasted amazing, like nothing we had ever experienced before. It was alive and nourishing. We were so happy to give our money to the farmers that actually grew it. We were supporting something we could believe in. It all started to make sense.

That was it, we were hooked. There was no turning back. We knew as we furthered our career in food, that it was about nourishing people from the inside out, it was about supporting the local economy, and eating foods close to the earth. We made the conscious choice to make this one of the foundations of our restaurant. Jessica got her masters in holistic nutrition to get a better understanding of the science of the whole foods approach and healing through foods. Holistic means "whole body" and it influenced how we created menus and every aspect of the restaurants we ran, events we hosted, and how we lived our day-to-day lives.

Gone were the cupboards of salty snacks and cereals loaded with ingredients we didn't know how to pronounce, gone were the dairy products that contained additives and preservatives and chemicals to strip the molecules from nourishing fat cells. Our shelves became stocked with wholesome fats (see "Fat Is Fabulous," page 156) and farmfresh milk and yogurt that retained all the delicious taste and live digestive enzymes that help keep the gut healthy. We began eating local meats and vibrant vegetables grown either in our gardens or by local farmers.

We felt so satiated and energized and the pounds just melted off. We came back to our healthy natural weights in no time. We felt fabulous knowing we weren't ingesting pesticides and hormones when we chose organic whole foods and we weren't going to feed that to our guests or families either. We learned that whole foods are way more potent, hold a higher nutritional value, contain more antioxidants, and keep the immune system strong. Today we start with whole foods for all of our recipes and prepare them in ways that hold on to the nutritional benefits and in some cases actually increase the nutritional content (see "Why Is Fermentation All the Rage?" on page 40).

Food is the ultimate medicine: it can heal, prevent disease, and energize your body. Eating whole foods without pesticides and hormones. is a commitment to yourself and to your health of the planet. It's saying YES, you want to live a life of optimal health. For us, it is now the only way—we are forever grateful to the farmers.

Here are some fun ideas to help you stay connected with your vegetables:

◆ Join a CSA, or Community Supported Agriculture, an arrangement that is often available from local farms where you pay a set cost up front and in exchange for an array of seasonal fruits and vegetables every week. It encourages creativity because you never know exactly what you are going to get! Some farms offer dairy and meat shares as well.

◆ Grow your own! Even with just a small plot of soil you can grow a good amount of veggies. Kale is easy to grow, as are many greens and herbs. Pick some of your favorite vegetables and go for it! Gardening is fun, educational, and wildly nutritious for the whole family.

CAESAR SALAD WITH ROASTED CHICKPEAS

Our version of Classic Caesar dressing has been a staple for years. We love it as a dip for cold chicken, with raw veggies, on sandwiches, and of course as the salad dressing. We like to make it in bigger batches and stash it in the fridge so it's at the ready for snacking.

The Vegan version is a favorite at Shine restaurant. It is unique in the way that the dulse seaweed takes the place of the anchovy and the almonds create the silky texture traditionally provided by the eggs. Dulse has a salty, oceany flavor and helps cleanse the body of heavy metals and supports brain function and healthy thyroid function.

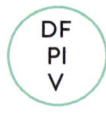

PI, DF (if using vegan dressing), V (if using classic dressing)

Serves 4 to 6

FOR THE CLASSIC CAESAR DRESSING (OR USE VEGAN CAESAR DRESSING, PAGE 69):

2 large soft-boiled eggs (page 20; see Tip)

¼ cup fresh lemon juice

3 cloves garlic, minced

¾ tablespoon anchovy paste (see Tip)

1 teaspoon Worcestershire sauce (check label to make sure it is gluten free)

½ teaspoon Dijon mustard

½ cup shredded Pecorino Romano cheese

1 cup extra-virgin olive oil

FOR THE SALAD

3 heads romaine hearts, torn into bite-sized pieces

¼ cup Roasted Chickpeas (page 68)

1. First make the dressing: Put all of the ingredients in a food processor except the olive oil and blend for 30 to 60 seconds. With the food processor running, slowly drizzle the olive oil down the chute to emulsify the dressing into a creamy consistency.

2. Put the romaine and roasted chickpeas in a salad bowl. Add the dressing and toss to coat.

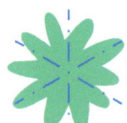

TIP

Feel free to get creative with your Caesar. We sometimes add crumbled bacon, soft-boiled egg, roasted tomatoes, or all three!

We like to soft-boil the eggs used in this dressing in order to make people feel comfortable with its safety and for their taste, but this dressing can also be made with raw pasteurized eggs. Anchovy is a strong flavor. You may want to start with less, then taste before your final mixing to see if you want add the full amount.

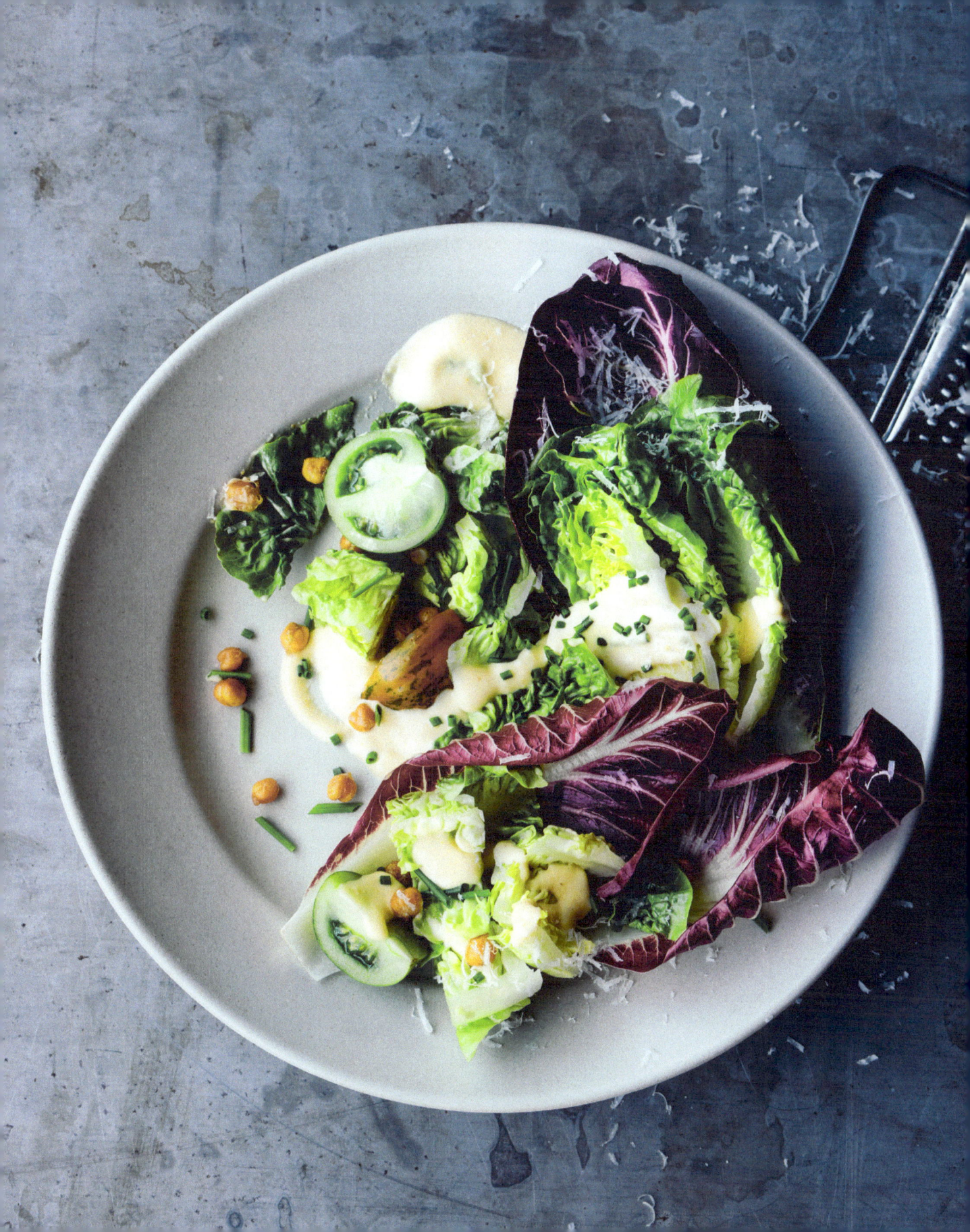

ROASTED CHICKPEAS

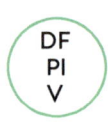

DF
PI
V

Chickpeas, otherwise known as garbanzo beans, are an Italian staple. Rich in fiber, they aid in digestion and help stabilize blood sugar. We added them to every salad while we were growing up. This is a more sophisticated version of that salad topper, and an alternative to croutons that also adds crunch and flavor.

Makes about 2 cups

2 cups cooked chickpeas (if using canned, choose a 15-ounce can)

2 tablespoons extra-virgin olive oil

½ teaspoon sea salt

1 teaspoon garlic powder

1. Preheat the oven to 400°F.

2. Rinse and drain the chickpeas in a strainer, place them on a clean kitchen towel, and pat them a few times to dry.

3. Whisk the olive oil, salt, and garlic powder together in a mixing bowl. Add the chickpeas and toss to coat. Spread them out evenly on a baking sheet.

4. Roast the chickpeas for 20 minutes. Gently shake the baking pan to move them around, and then bake them for another 5 minutes until lightly golden.

5. Serve straight out of the oven. The chickpeas will keep for up to 4 days at room temperature in a sealed container.

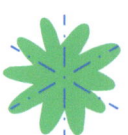

TIP

There are many different things you can do with the flavoring of these chickpeas. Some of our favorites are shaking on powdered curry or an Italian herb blend, or tossing the chickpeas in melted ghee and Pecorino Romano cheese

Jessica: My daughter Amelie loves snacking on these chickpeas after school and before her swim practice for a salty (and healthy) fix.

VEGAN CAESAR DRESSING

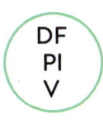

DF
PI
V

Put all of the ingredients except for the oil in a blender and run it for 1 minute. With the blender running, slowly drizzle in the olive oil for a creamy finish.

Makes about 2½ cups

1 cup blanched (skinless) almonds (see Tip), soaked for 3 hours or simmered for 20 minutes

1¼ cups water

2 cloves garlic, peeled

¾ cup fresh lemon juice

1 tablespoon plus 1 teaspoon dulse seaweed flakes

¼ cup nutritional yeast

2 teaspoons Dijon mustard

1 tablespoon capers plus 2 teaspoons of the brine

1 teaspoon sea salt

¾ cup extra-virgin olive oil

TIP

Blanched almonds work the best in this recipe. If you can't find them in the store, blanching natural almonds to remove their skins is an easy process. Begin by bringing a small pot of water to a boil. Place the almonds in the water for exactly 1 minute. If you boil them any longer, the almonds will become too soft. Drain the almonds in a colander and rinse under cold water to cool them. Blot them with a paper towel and use your fingers to gently squeeze the almonds to loosen and remove the skins.

ARUGULA, PEAR AND BLUE CHEESE SALAD WITH HONEY WALNUT VINAIGRETTE

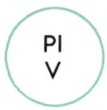

PI
V

When using blue cheeses, note that not all of them are gluten-free. If this concerns you, check the packaging to be sure. The walnuts in the dressing add flavor, texture, and a protein boost.

Serves 4 to 6

FOR THE
HONEY WALNUT
VINAIGRETTE

½ cup walnut pieces

2 tablespoons minced shallots

¼ cup red wine vinegar

1 tablespoon raw honey

½ teaspoon dried thyme (optional)

1 cup extra-virgin olive oil

¼ cup water

Sea salt to taste

FOR THE SALAD

2 cups baby arugula

½ cup crumbled blue cheese

¾ cup skinned, diced pear

¼ cup chopped dates

1. First make the dressing: Put all in the blender except for the olive oil and water and blend thoroughly. While still blending, slowly add the olive oil. Add the water slowly to get the desired consistency. You may not need all of it. Add salt to taste.

2. Put all of the salad ingredients in a large bowl and toss with the Honey Walnut Vinaigrette to coat.

TIP

In the winter time it could be hard to find arugula but you can sub it out with another spicy green like spinach or simple mixed greens.

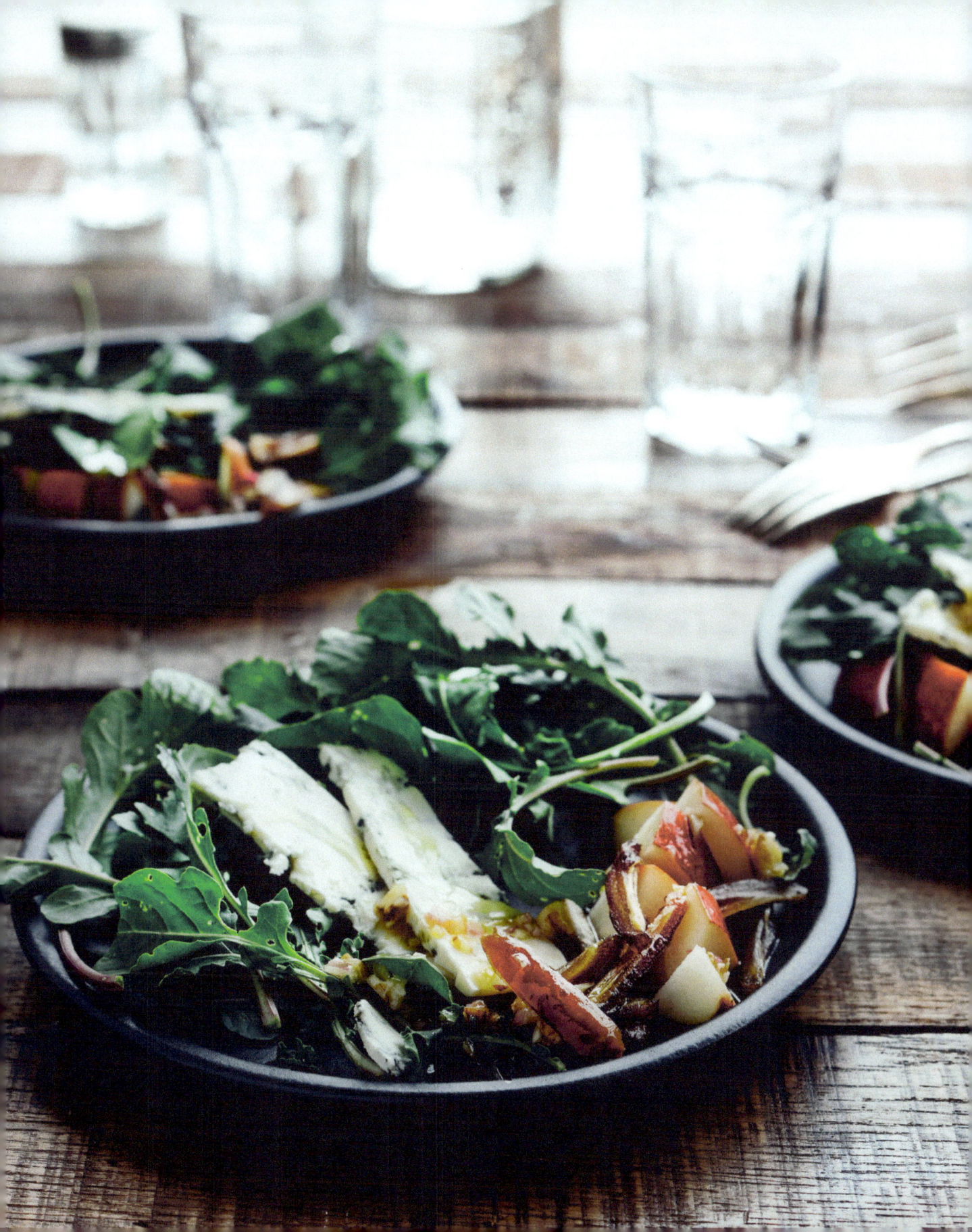

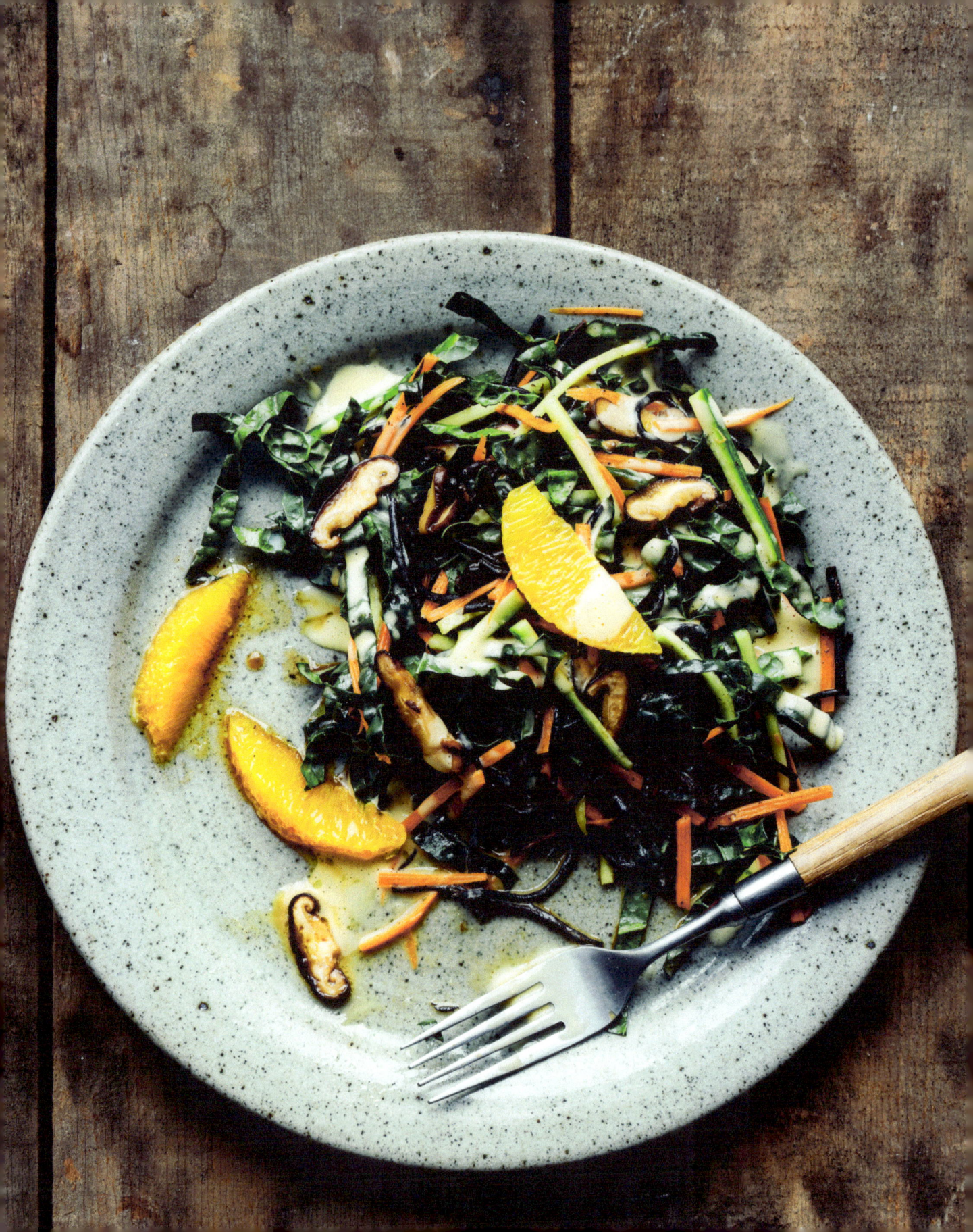

KALE AND HIJIKI SALAD WITH ORANGE TAHINI DRESSING

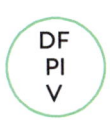

DF
PI
V

Hijiki is a type of seaweed. Some of the greatest health benefits are balancing hormonal activity, improved energy levels, and strengthening for bones. This salad is a powerhouse of nutrition and delivers in flavor. Pan-seared Fish (page 84) or chicken (page 86) is a great addition to this salad.

Serves 3 to 4

¼ cup hijiki seaweed

½ cup sliced shiitake mushrooms, stems removed

1 tablespoon extra-virgin olive oil

1½ teaspoons gluten-free tamari

2 cups shredded kale leaves

1 cup shredded carrots

1 cup peeled julienned cucumbers

2 tablespoons sesame seeds, for garnish (optional)

½ cup Orange Tahini Dressing (recipe below

1. Rinse the hijiki, cover with water, and soak for 20 to 30 minutes until tender. Drain, rinse, and set aside.

2. Meanwhile, in a mixing bowl, toss the shiitakes with the olive oil and tamari. Marinate for 15 minutes.

3. To the bowl of marinated mushrooms, add the kale, carrots, cucumbers, and sesame seeds, along with the drained hijiki. Drizzle the salad with the dressing and toss to coat. Serve immediately.

ORANGE TAHINI DRESSING

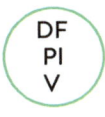

DF
PI
V

Combine all of the ingredients in a blender and blend for 1 minute until creamy. Store in an airtight container in the refrigerator for up to 5 days.

Makes about 2 cups

1 cup orange juice

⅓ cup raw tahini (sesame seed paste)

½ cup extra-virgin olive oil

¼ cup avocado oil

1 teaspoon apple cider vinegar

1 teaspoon tamari

sea salt to taste

TIP

Tahini can be expensive. You can easily make your own by blending 1 cup sesame seeds with 2 tablespoons mild olive oil or sesame oil. This homemade tahini can be stored for up to 1 month in the refrigerator.

CHOPPED GARDEN SALAD WITH DAIRY-FREE RANCH

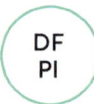

**DF
PI**

Ranch is one of the most popular—and least healthy—dressings out there. Our dairy-free version is a fantastic alternative that makes a wonderful salad dressing, dip for chips and vegetables, as well as a sauce for fish sticks (page 92) and chicken fingers (page 97).

Serves 4 to 6

FOR THE DAIRY-FREE RANCH DRESSING:

½ cup mayonnaise, store-bought or homemade (page 90)

½ cup full-fat canned coconut milk

1 teaspoon raw apple cider vinegar

2 teaspoons chopped fresh dill

1 tablespoon chopped fresh chives

1 teaspoon chopped fresh parsley

½ teaspoon onion powder

¼ teaspoon gluten-free Worcestershire sauce

Sea salt to taste

FOR THE SALAD:

I head romaine lettuce, chopped into bite-sized pieces

2 cups mixed greens

¾ cup halved cherry tomatoes

1 avocado, halved, pitted, and diced

1 cup diced cucumbers

2 tablespoons sliced red onion

2 hard-boiled eggs, peeled and chopped

2 tablespoons chopped cooked bacon

1. First make the dressing: Whisk all of the ingredients together in a mixing bowl. Season with salt. Store in an airtight container in the refrigerator for up to 5 days.

2. Toss all of the ingredients in a salad bowl. Add the Dairy-free Ranch Dressing, toss to coat, and serve..

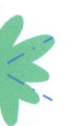 **TIP**

You can play with different herbs and spices to create different flavors for the many ways you will use this dressing.

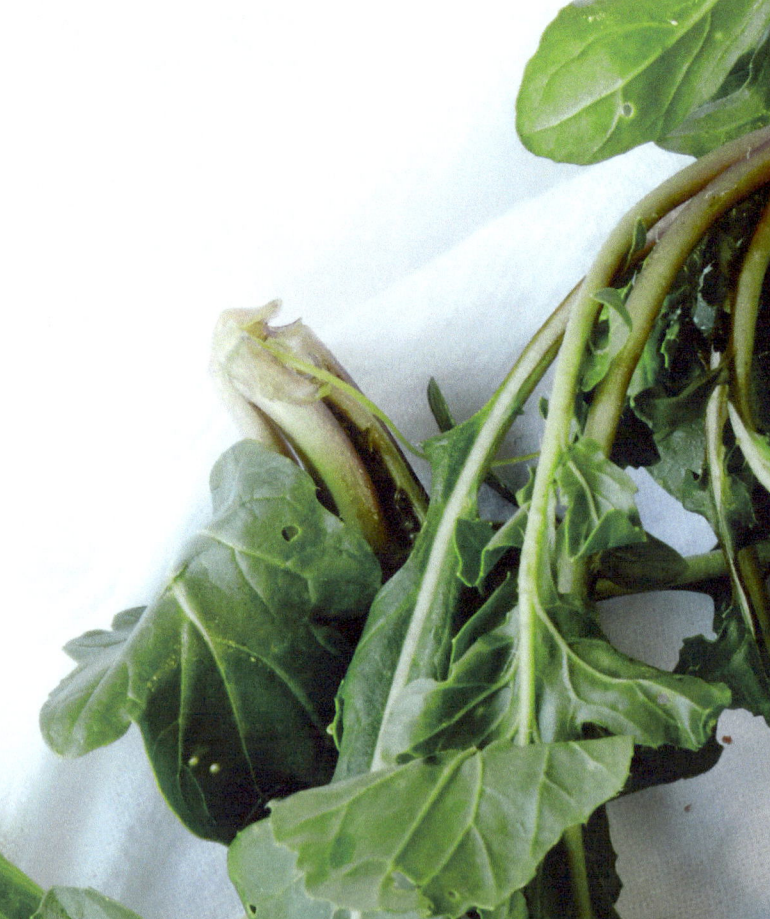

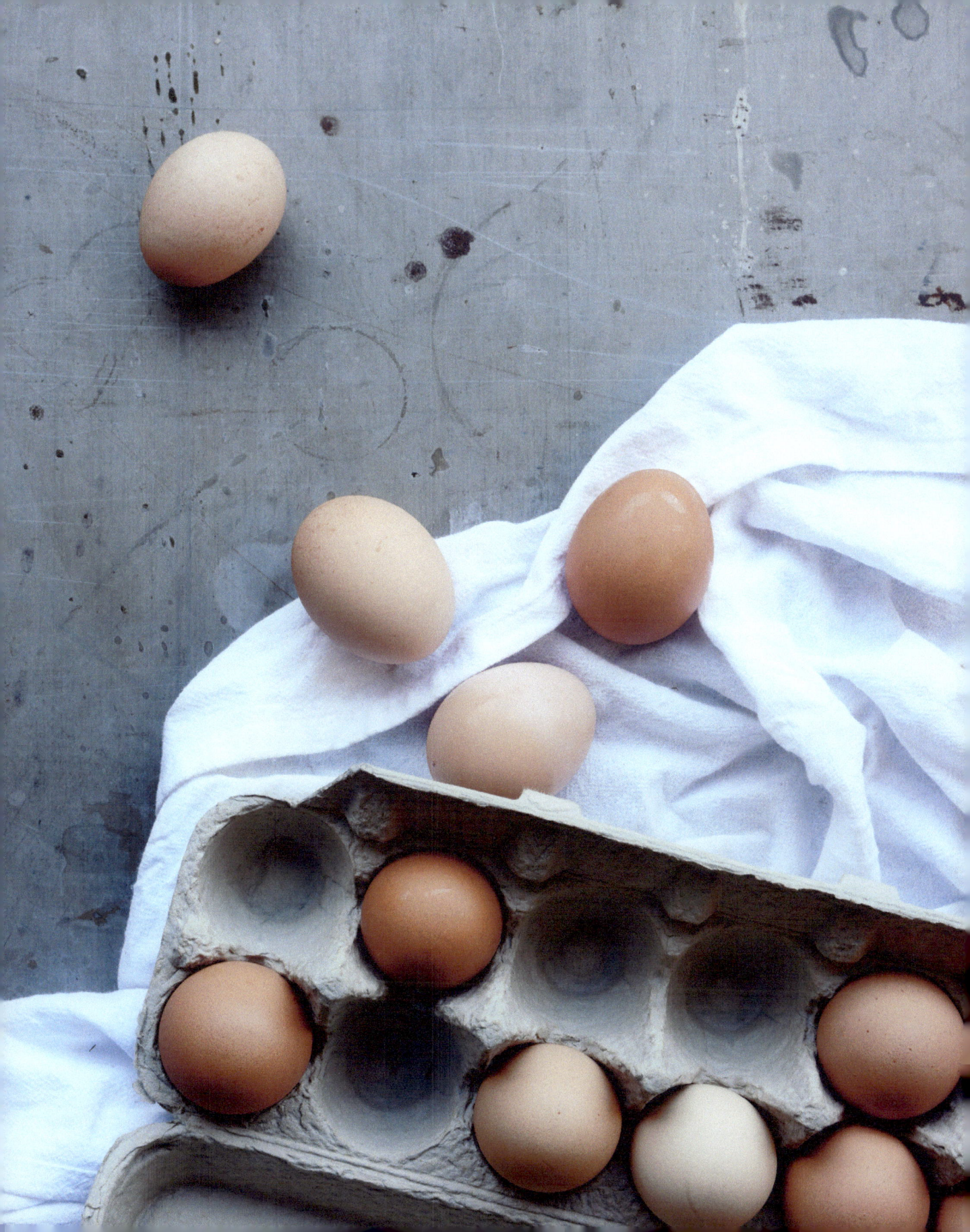

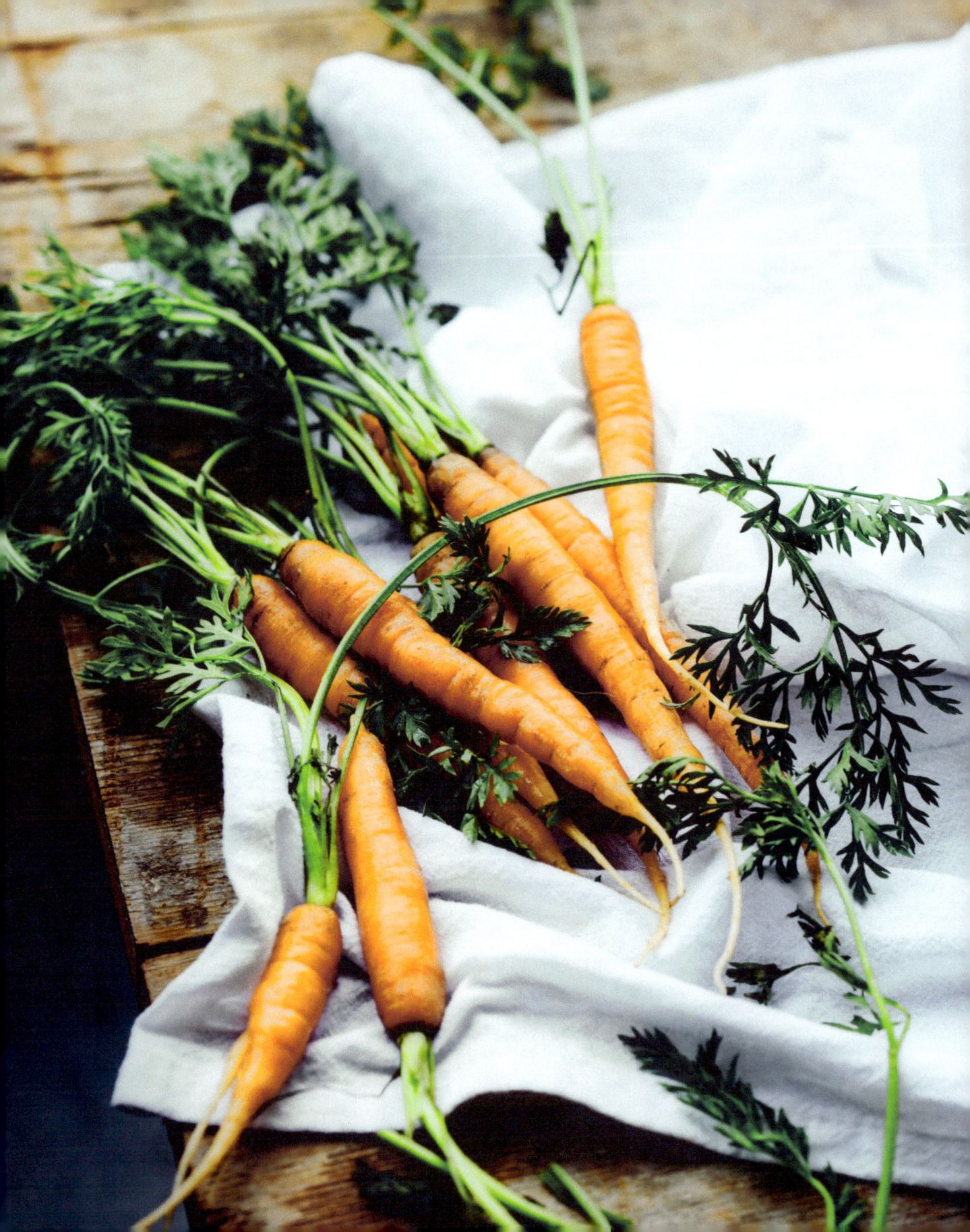

MIXED GREEN SALAD WITH SPROUTED SUNFLOWER SEED VINAIGRETTE

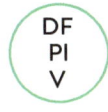

DF
PI
V

Serves 4 to 6

FOR THE SPROUTED
SUNFLOWER SEED
VINAIGRETTE:

¾ cup raw, hulled, whole
sunflower seeds, soaked in
3 cups water for 6 hours
or overnight (see Tip)

1 clove garlic

½ tablespoon peeled,
minced fresh ginger

1 tablespoon minced
fresh lemongrass
or 1 teaspoon dried
powdered lemongrass

¾ cup distilled water

¼ cup light miso paste

¾ cup olive extra-
virgin olive oil

1 tablespoon fresh
lemon juice

Sea salt to taste

FOR THE SALAD:

5 cups mixed greens

½ cup shredded carrots

½ cup halved and
thinly sliced radishes

½ cup thinly sliced
cucumbers

1. First make the dressing. Drain and rinse the sunflower seeds and put them in a high-powered blender. Add the garlic, ginger, and lemongrass and run the blender for 1 minute. Add the distilled water and run for 30 seconds. Add the miso paste and lemon juice and run for 1 minute more. While the blender is running, slowly add the olive oil. Check the vinaigrette for salt. It may not need it depending on the saltiness of the miso.

2. Toss the greens and vegetables together in a salad bowl. Add the vinaigrette and toss to coat.

TIP

This is a simple green salad. What makes it special is the vinaigrette.

The sprouted sunflower seeds called for in this recipe are at the beginning of the sprouting process. You can take it further by returning the drained and rinsed seeds to the soaking container without water to sit for another 6 to 8 hours. This will create a more pronounced sprout with a light, artichoke-like flavor. Very often we soak the sprouted sunflower seeds like this, just to add them to salads on their own. After sprouting, they will keep for up to 5 days in the refrigerator.

Jessica: When I figured out that sprouting sunflower seeds and then pureeing them would create a creamy dressing, I was thrilled! It opened up a whole new world. I love the consistency of this dressing. It is flavorful and creamy. I know it may sound like a lot to soak seeds for a dressing you are making the next day, but it is actually very simple and your belly will thank you.

RED CABBAGE AND SWEET CARROT SLAW WITH GINGER VINAIGRETTE

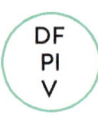

DF
PI
V

There is a lot of grating required, which makes this recipe a bit of a workout for the biceps, so roll up your sleeves and get into it. What does make it convenient though, is that it keeps for several days, even if it's already dressed.

Serves 4 to 6

FOR THE GINGER VINAIGRETTE:

2 tablespoons peeled, minced fresh ginger

2 teaspoons minced garlic

3 tablespoons toasted sesame oil

¼ cup gluten-free tamari

3 tablespoons fresh lime juice

2 teaspoons raw honey

FOR THE SALAD:

½ head large red cabbage, cored and thinly sliced

½ head broccoli, stem removed, grated or shredded in a food processor

1 carrot, grated

4 radishes, halved and thinly sliced

1 tablespoon sesame seeds

1. First make the dressing: Put the ingredients in a small bowl and whisk them together.

2. Put all of the vegetables in a large bowl. Add the Ginger Vinaigrette and toss to coat the salad well. Garnish with the sesame seeds, wipe your brow, and serve.

TIP

This is the ultimate potluck salad because it goes well with just about anything, both hot or cold, and people love it.

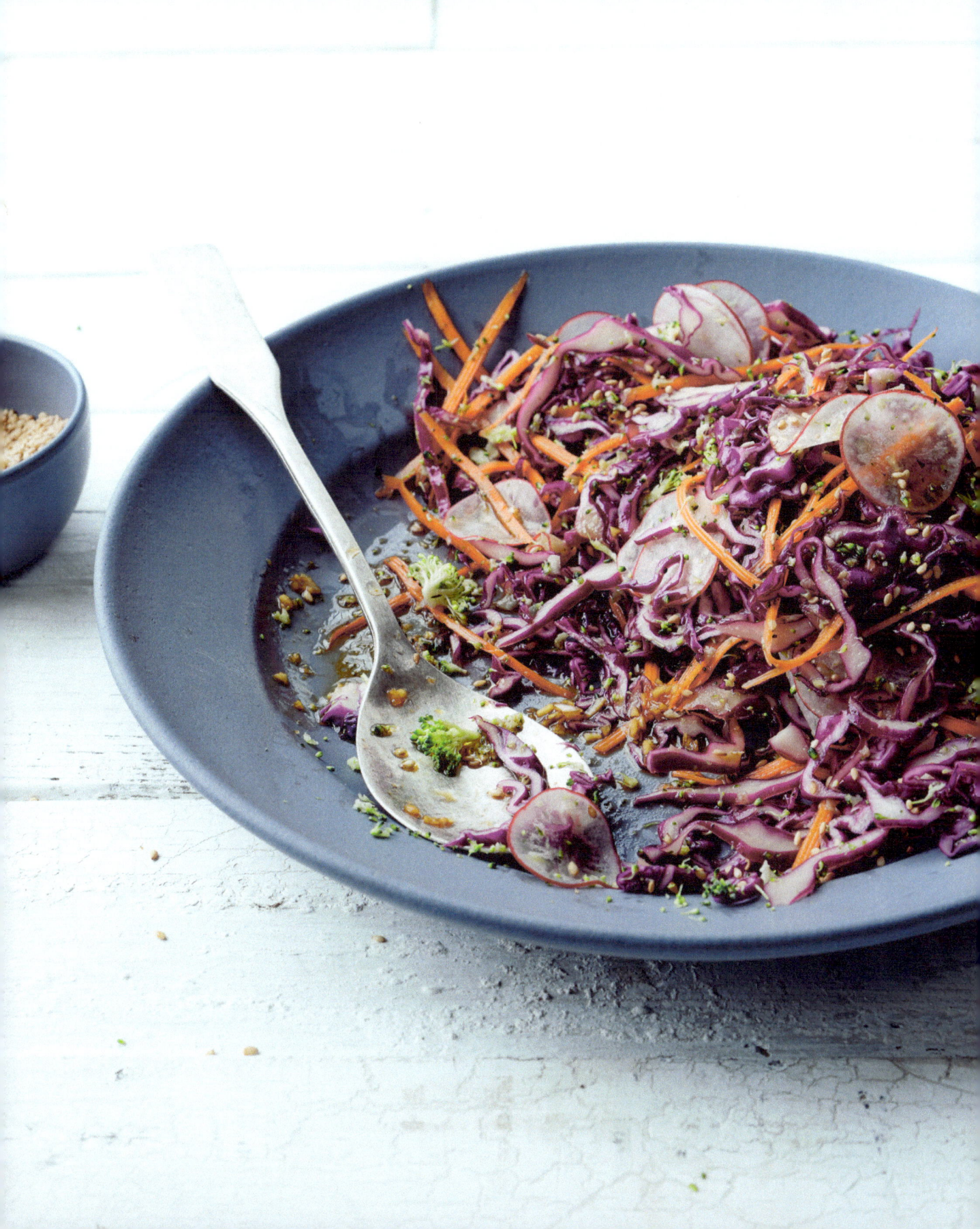

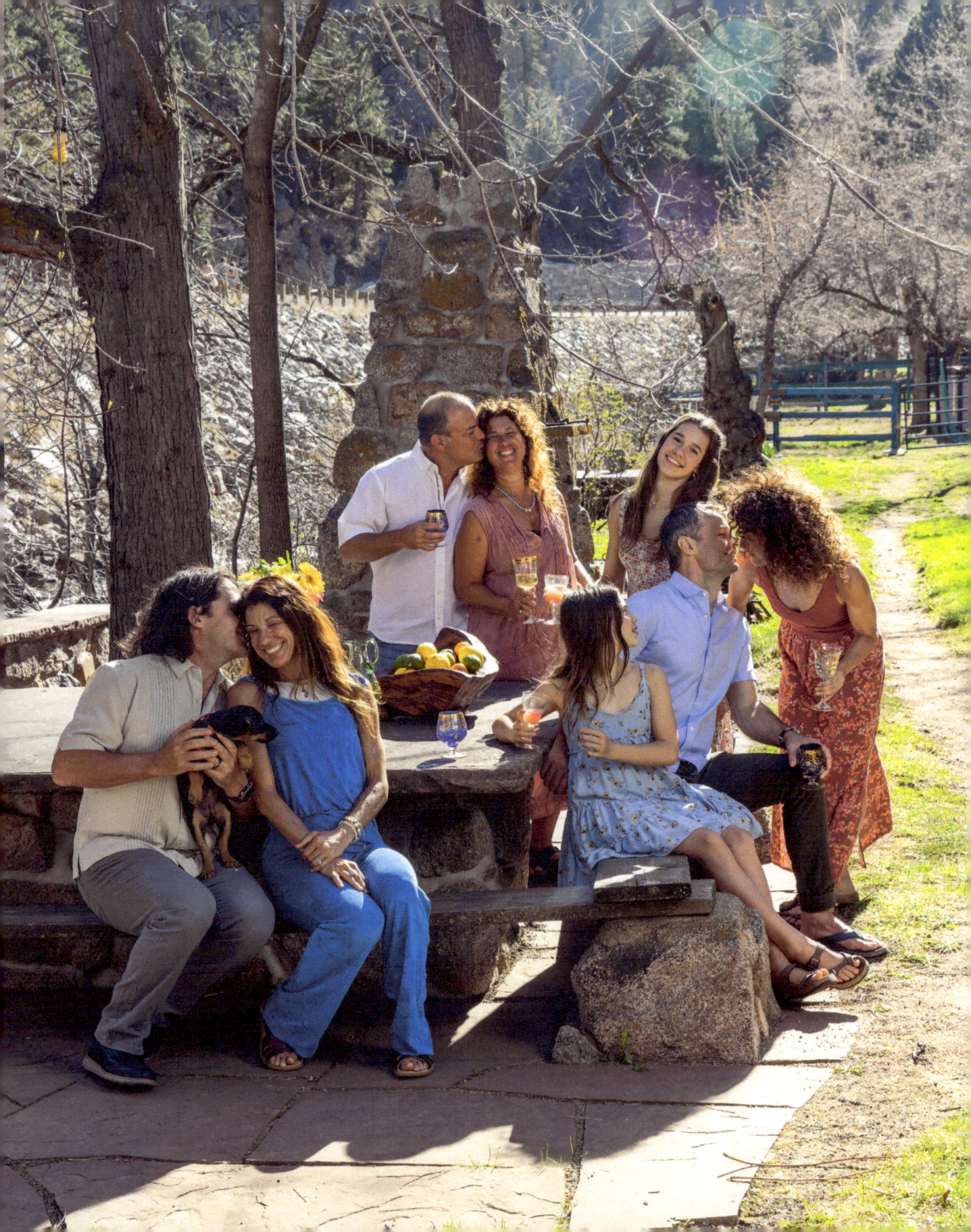

EASY-BREEZY MASSAGED KALE & AVOCADO SALAD

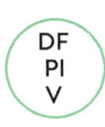

DF
PI
V

Kale is so beautiful and so healthy, and yet some people find that eating it can feel like a lot of work. This recipe makes it tender, delicious, and easy for the whole family to enjoy. Massaging the kale with lemon juice makes it easy to digest, so all of the vitamins and minerals are readily available to your body.

Serves 4 to 6

2 bunches curly kale (Tuscan or dinosaur)

¼ cup fresh lemon juice

2 to 3 teaspoons sea salt

1 ripe avocado, pitted, peeled, and diced

3 tablespoons extra-virgin olive oil

1. Remove the ribs from the kale and cut the leaves into bite-sized pieces. Put the leaves in a large mixing bowl.

2. Add the lemon juice, sea salt, avocado, and olive oil to the kale. Get all up and personal with the kale, massaging it thoroughly to distribute the ingredients with your hands for approximately 10 minutes, until the leaves soften, darken in color, shrink in size, and become a silky texture. (You may want to remove your jewelry for this part!)

3. Let the salad sit for approximately 20 minutes before serving to let all the flavors sink in.

TIP

Add your favorite salad add-ons, such as seared chicken, steak, or fish to make this a meal in a bowl.

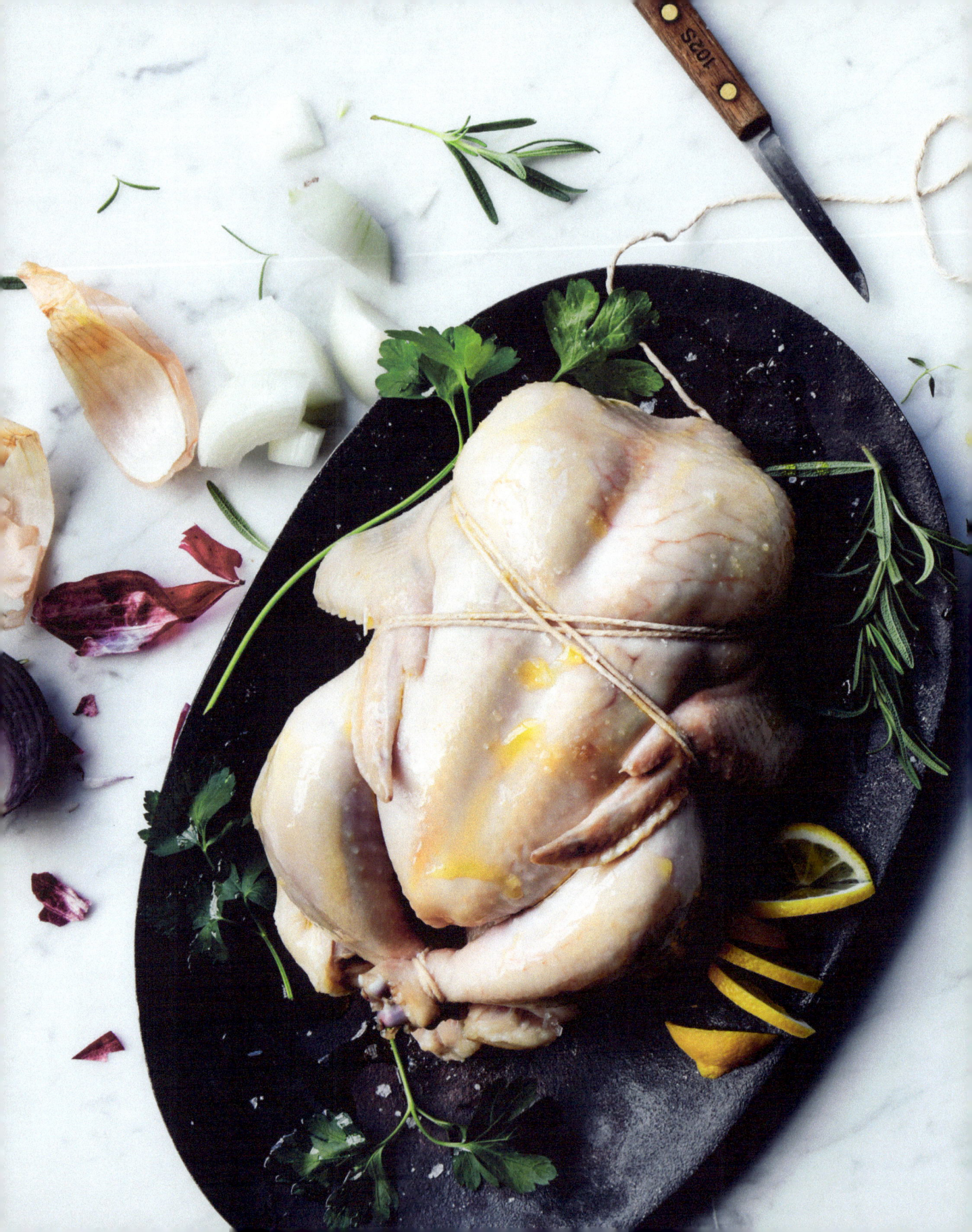

MEAT, FISH & POULTRY

Protein is an important part of any diet. The easiest way to get it is from nutritionally dense proteins like meat, fish, and poultry, as well as eggs, nuts, and seeds. Without enough protein, you can feel fatigued and your brainpower might be turned on to low volume. The quality of the meat you choose is important to getting the proper nutrients into your diet, too. See our sourcing page (page 113).

"Find your hero's journey and light up the path."

PAN-SEARED FISH WITH CRISPY SKIN

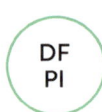

**DF
PI**

Even in landlocked Boulder, Colorado, we love fish and can locally source a variety of lake trout. Find a fish that is available wild or sustainably farmed in your area. Serve these crisp-skinned fillets on top of salads, as a main feature to a vegetable dish, or with your favorite style of eggs. We like the acidity of lemon or lime to add some piquant flavor.

Serves 4 to 6

4 to 6 fish fillets, about 5-ounces each, skin on and bones out (salmon, bass, trout, or snapper)

2 tablespoons unsalted butter, ghee, coconut oil, or extra-virgin olive oil

Sea salt to taste

1 lemon, sliced, for serving

1. Using a sharp knife to score the skin side of each fillet with shallow incisions, not piercing the flesh. This will help prevent the skin from curling up.

2. Heat a large cast-iron skillet or sauté pan to medium to high heat. Add the fat to the pan (we prefer ghee) and salt both sides of the fish just before searing it.

3. Add the fish to the hot pan, skin side down, and let the skin crisp up and the flesh cook about two thirds of the way through, 3 to 5 minutes, depending on the thickness. You can baste the fish with the fat as it is cooking, but do not move it until it is ready to be flipped. (Coax it with a spatula to see if it is ready.)

4. Once the fish is cooked most of the way through and the skin is brown and crispy, flip the fish using a spatula. Cook flesh side down until just cooked through. This should only take a minute or two (see Tip).

5. Serve immediately with lemon slices to garnish.

TIP

Keep an eye on the fish as you cook it, as overcooked fish loses its delicate flavor and can become more "fishy" tasting and dry.

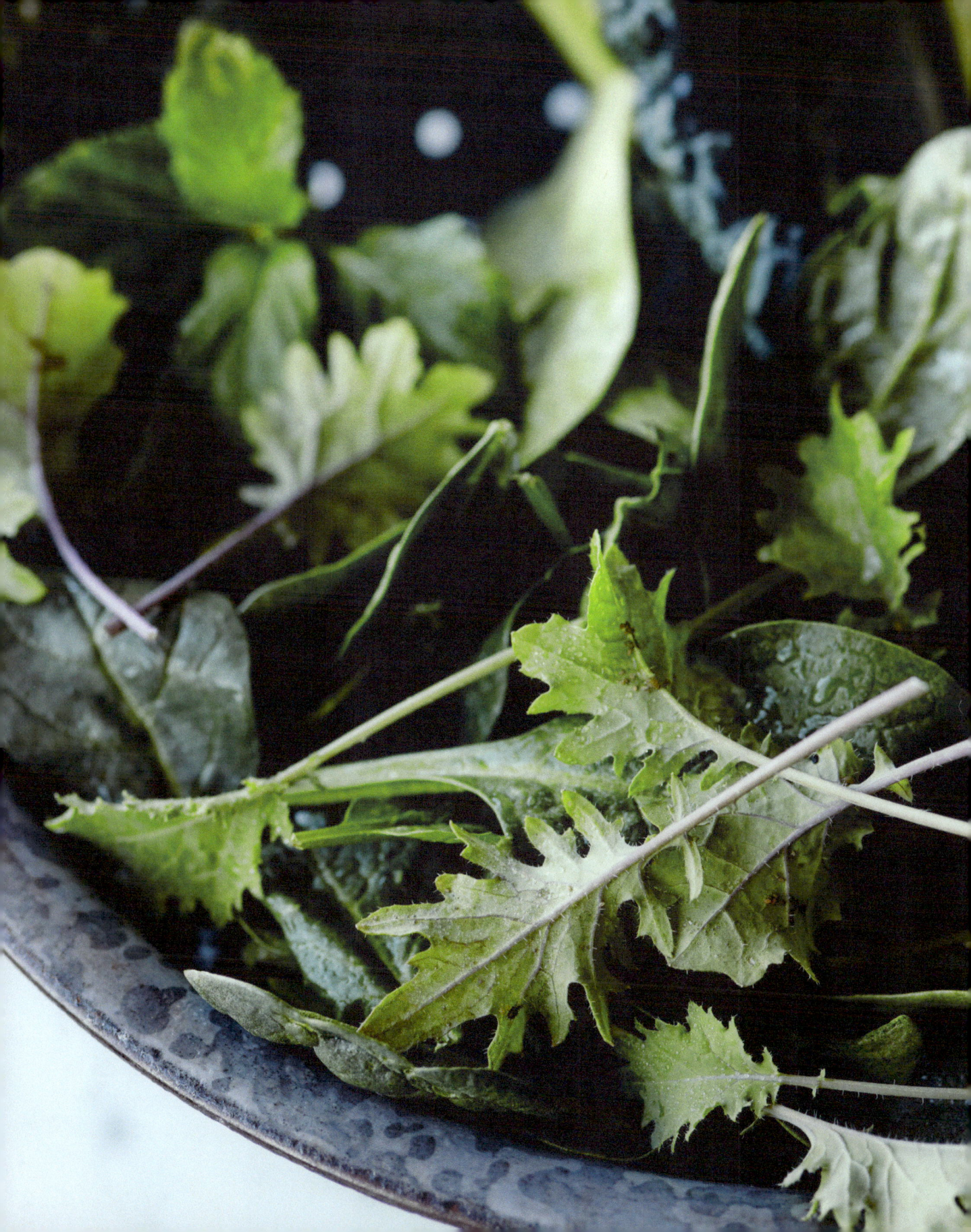

PAN-SEARED BONE-IN CHICKEN THIGHS

Properly searing chicken is a good technique to know for quick meals and as an addition to salads. You can use dark meat or breasts. We prefer the legs and thighs because of their flavor and texture. We love to serve the leftovers cold for lunch the next day, over greens or on their own.

DF
PI

Serves 4 to 6

4 to 6 bone-in, skin-on free-range chicken thighs

Sea salt to taste

2 tablespoons extra-virgin olive oil

1. Preheat the oven to 425°F.

2. Generously season the chicken on both sides with salt.

3. Heat a large cast-iron skillet or sauté pan to medium-high. Add the olive oil. Put the chicken in the hot pan, skin side down. Let the skin crisp up and brown, 4 to 6 minutes.

4. Flip the chicken so it is flesh side down in the pan and let it cook for another 4 to 6 minutes, until lightly browned. Turn off the heat.

5. Cover the skillet with aluminum foil and bake for 20 to 25 minutes. The chicken is done when it reaches an internal temperature of 165°F on a meat thermometer.

6. Let the chicken sit for 5 minutes before serving.

TIP
You can pan-sear breasts this way as well; just cut the oven-baking time to 10 to 12 minutes.

PAN-SEARED STEAK

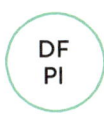

DF
PI

We cook our meat to medium-rare, meaning pink on the inside. We find that the flavor and tenderness is best this way. In addition, it keeps some live enzymes intact to make the meat easier on your digestive system. This rosemary and garlic seasoned steak is great as a salad topper, alongside vegetable sides, or for a hearty steak and eggs breakfast.

Serves 4 to 6

4 to 6 grass-fed steaks (rib-eye, flat-iron, strip, or tenderloin), about 5 ounces per person

Sea salt to taste

¼ cup extra-virgin olive oil

½ tablespoon fresh rosemary, chopped

½ tablespoon chopped shallots (optional)

½ teaspoon chopped garlic (optional)

1 tablespoon unsalted butter (optional)

1. Salt steaks generously, ideally about 30 minutes before cooking.

2. Heat a large cast-iron skillet or sauté pan to medium to high heat. Add the olive oil. Sear the steaks until they are a deep golden brown, then flip them and sear on the other side, 4 to 5 minutes per side. Lower the heat to medium and cook the steaks until golden brown.

3. While the steak is cooking, add the rosemary to the pan along with the shallots and garlic, if using. If you are using the butter, add it to the pan, too, and baste the steak by spooning the butter over the steak. Cook the steak until medium rare or desired temperature (see Tip).

4. Let the steak rest for 5 to 10 minutes to allow the juices to settle to maintain the moistness and flavor. Serve with a side of vegetables or a salad.

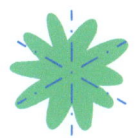

TIP

To cook the steak to your desired doneness, use a meat thermometer to measure the internal temperature:

Rare: 120°F
Medium-rare (perfect): 130°F
Medium: 140°F
Medium well: 150°F
Well: 160°F

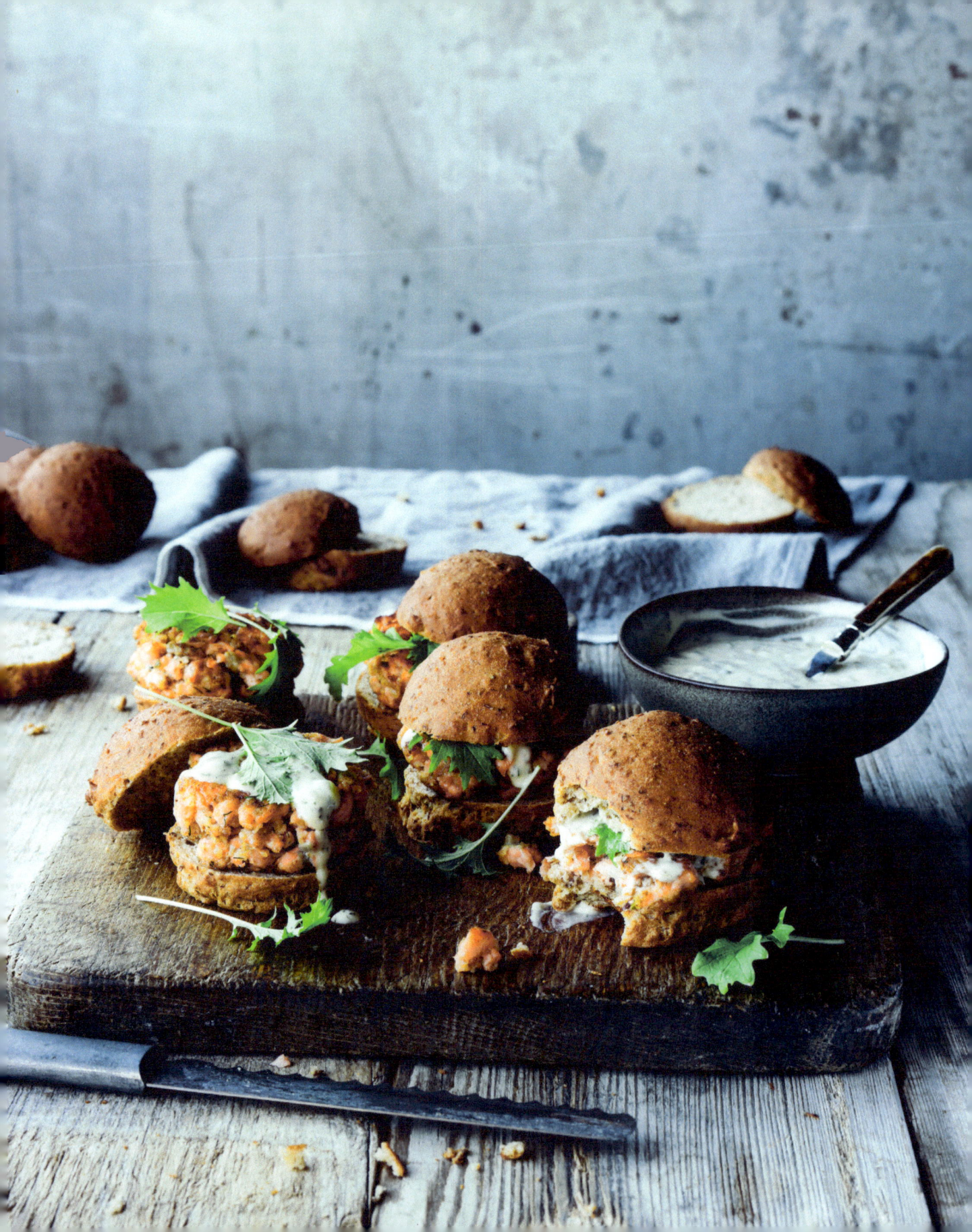

SALMON BURGER PATTIES

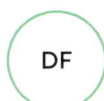

DF

It's fun to change up your usual burger by using salmon instead of beef. Creating your own salmon burgers makes them more economical, plus you can get creative with the flavors. These tend to cook up the best in a sauté pan, but they do also work well on the grill. Choosing sustainably farmed or wild salmon supports the proper treatment of seafood, and it is high in healthful fats.

Makes eight 4-ounce servings

2 pounds wild or sustainably farmed salmon fillets, skin and bones removed, cut into small dice

½ tablespoon capers, drained and finely chopped

2 tablespoons Whole-Egg Mayonnaise (page 90) or storebought mayo

1 tablespoon fresh lemon juice

1 cup Gluten-Free Breadcrumbs (page 91)

1 tablespoon minced shallots

1 tablespoon finely chopped fresh dill

Sea salt to taste

2 to 3 tablespoons coconut oil

1. Put the diced salmon in large mixing bowl. Add the capers, mayonnaise, lemon juice, breadcrumbs, shallots, and dill. Add a pinch of salt and mix well.

2. Using a half-cup measuring cup, divide the salmon mixture into 8 portions and form into patties.

3. Heat a large sauté pan on medium and then melt enough of the coconut oil to cover the bottom of the pan.

4. When the oil is hot, put 2 to 4 patties in the pan, depending on the size of your pan. Cook for approximately 5 minutes before flipping the patties over. (Carefully test with a spatula to see if you can lift the burgers without sticking. If they are not easy to lift, wait another minute or two or add a little more oil.) Cook for 5 minutes on the other side, or until lightly browned. Transfer to a platter.

5. Add more coconut oil to the pan, if needed, and cook the remaining patties.

6. Serve these patties on a bed of arugula with lemon wedges and/or on a bun with our Tartar Sauce (page 93) or Sunflower Arugula Pesto (page 40).

TIP

Because fresh wild salmon is not available year-round, sometimes we buy it frozen. These salmon patties work out well when made with previously frozen wild salmon.

WHOLE-EGG MAYONNAISE

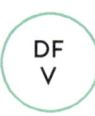

DF
V

We love mayo! Growing up we enjoyed a lot of mayo on our sandwiches and even used it as a dipper for cold chicken or turkey. It is easy to make and can be a healthy addition to your diet. With this recipe you avoid additives, preservatives, and unhealthy oils that are in many of the store-bought varieties.

Makes about 2 cups

1 whole egg plus 1 egg yolk, both at room temperature

1 tablespoon Dijon mustard

2 teaspoons sherry vinegar or white wine vinegar

1 tablespoon fresh lemon juice

1¾ cups extra-virgin olive oil or avocado oil

1. Add the egg and yolk, mustard, vinegar, and lemon juice to a high-powered blender or food processor. Blend for 30 seconds.

2. With the blender or food processor running, very slowly begin to drizzle in the oil (a very slow drip is what's required here). Continue to add drip by drip until the mixture starts to emulsify and thicken. At this point, you can begin to pour the oil a bit faster until the mixture reaches a mayonnaise consistency. As soon as you have a mayonnaise consistency, stop processing.

3. The mayonnaise can be used immediately or refrigerated in a glass container for up to 5 days.

TIP

Mayonnaise can be flavored in many different ways depending on how you are going to use it. We blend in roasted garlic, sun-dried tomatoes, or basil pesto to name a few of our favorites.

HOMEMADE GLUTEN-FREE BREADCRUMBS

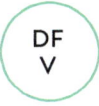

DF
V

Store-bought gluten-free breadcrumbs can be pricey. Why spend the money when they are so easy to make at home from leftover bread?

4 to 5 slices gluten-free bread, any kind

½ teaspoon kosher salt (optional)

Dried seasonings, such as oregano and parsley to taste (optional)

1. Preheat the oven to 325°F.

2. Bake the bread on a baking sheet until dry and toasted, about 8 to 10 minutes, flipping over once while baking; let cool completely. Alternatively, dry out the bread on the counter, uncovered, overnight.

3. Break up the slices of dried bread into chunks, place in a food processor, and pulse until coarse crumbs form. Add the optional salt and seasonings, if using, and pulse again until combined, or until the crumbs reach the desired consistency. (We prefer coarser panko-style crumbs, but you may like to grind them fine.)

4. Transfer the breadcrumbs to the prepared baking sheet and bake on the center rack for another 5 to 10 minutes, stirring occasionally.

5. Cool on the baking sheet before transferring the crumbs to a freezer-safe container. Seal tightly and store in the refrigerator or freezer until ready to use.

TIP

The crumbs can be used directly from the refrigerator or freezer, without defrosting, and will stay fresh in the refrigerator for about 5 days and for months in the freezer.

FISH STICKS WITH TARTAR SAUCE

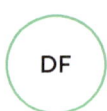

DF

This crunchy finger food is a good way to get kids eating fish. Not only are they fun for dipping, they contain Omega-3s, which help brain development. Even the fish-averse adults in your life will enjoy these, especially with our creamy tartar sauce for dipping.

Serves 4 to 6

1 ½ pounds firm white fish that is skinned and deboned (we prefer cod)

½ cup brown rice flour

1 teaspoon sea salt

3 large eggs

2 cups Gluten-Free Breadcrumbs (page 91)

2 tablespoons extra-virgin olive oil

4 to 5 tablespoons coconut oil

Sea salt to taste

Tartar Sauce (page 93), for serving

Lemon wedges, for garnish

1. Prepare your ingredients and arrange them in the following sequence near your stovetop: Cut the fish into wide strips, about 1 x 3 inches each. Mix the flour and salt on a large flat plate. Whisk the eggs in a large bowl. Mix the breadcrumbs and olive oil in another large bowl.

2. Individually coat each strip of fish in the flour mixture and set aside on a plate. When all of the fish is coated with flour, dip each piece individually in the egg wash, and then coat thoroughly in the breadcrumbs; set aside on a plate.

3. Heat a large sauté pan on medium-high. Add half of the coconut oil to the pan. When the oil is completely melted, place some of the coated fish strips in the pan. (Do not overcrowd the pan—you will need to cook in batches.) Cook for a few minutes on each side, until the fish strips have a nice golden brown color. Transfer them to a paper-towel-lined plate to drain. Repeat this step with the remaining coconut oil and fish sticks.

4. Serve the fish sticks hot with tartar sauce and lemon wedges.

TIP

Mayonnaise can be flavored in many different ways depending on how you are going to use it. We blend in roasted garlic, sun-dried tomatoes, or basil pesto to name a few of our favorites.

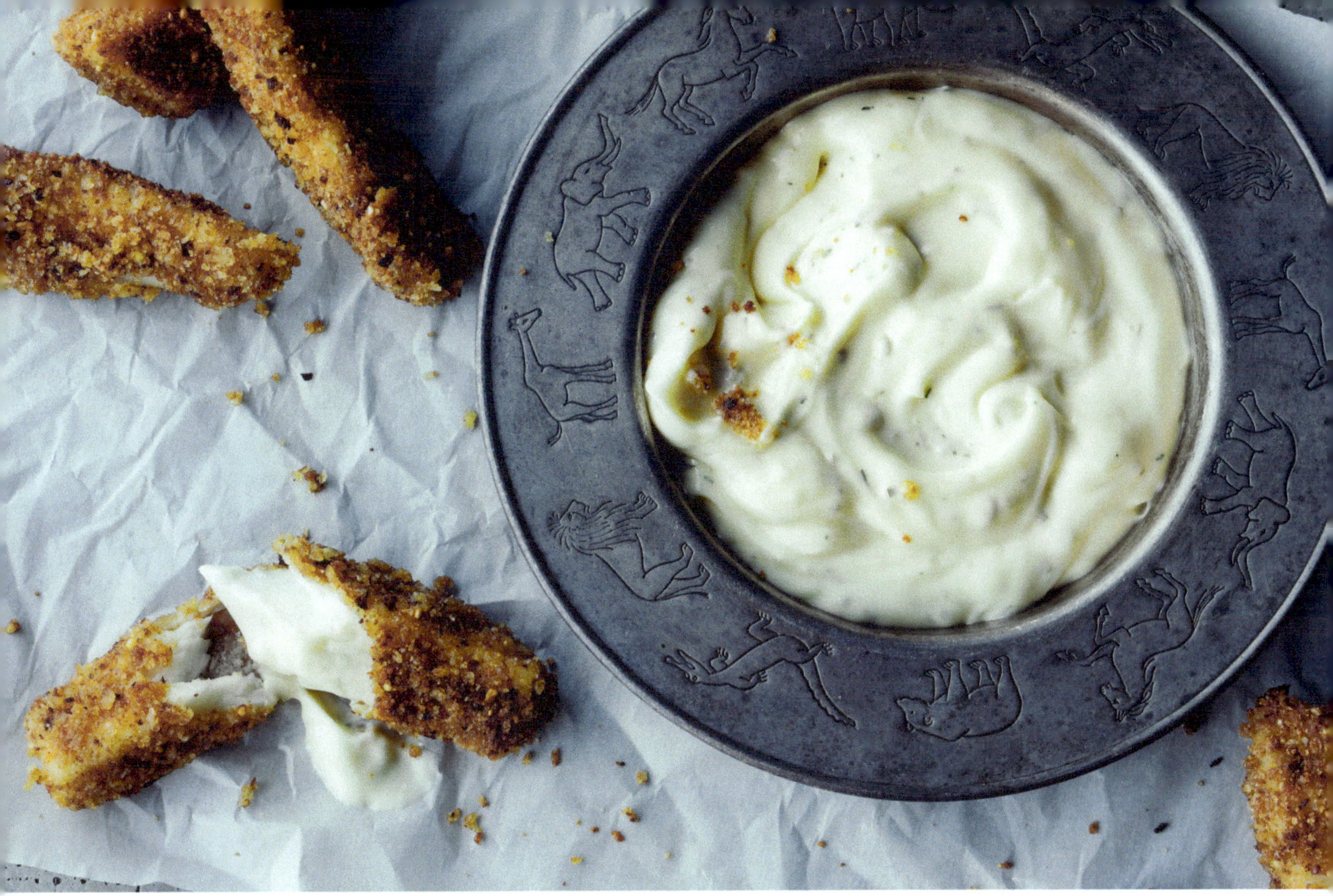

TANGY TARTAR SAUCE

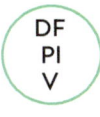

This tangy sauce is a natural accompaniment to fish. It is fresh tasting and adds vibrancy and acidity to play beautifully as a spread or dipping sauce.

Makes about 1 cup

¾ cup Whole-Egg Mayonnaise (page 90) or store-bought

3 tablespoons finely diced pickles

1 tablespoon chopped capers

1 tablespoon chopped fresh dill

2 teaspoons fresh lemon juice

1 teaspoon raw apple cider vinegar

Sea salt to taste

Stir together all of the ingredients in a mixing bowl. Store in an airtight container in the refrigerator for up to 5 days.

SEAFOOD STEW WITH BASIL PESTO

This is always part of our annual Christmas Eve family dinner. Our grand-mother loved to make it with calamari and serve it over homemade pasta. There are many different kinds of seafood you can use here, so ask your fish guy what is looking the best. This stew is versatile enough to serve as a fancy dinner or a simple meal. Present it over pasta, or serve it with warm, crusty gluten-free bread and your favorite bottle of wine.

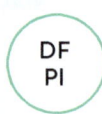
DF
PI

Serves 4 to 6

2 tablespoons extra-virgin olive oil

1 small onion, chopped

1 teaspoon fennel seeds

2 teaspoons dried oregano

2 cloves garlic, minced

½ pound cleaned calamari, cut into ½-inch rings (see Tip)

½ pound salmon fillets, skinned, boned, and diced into small pieces

1 cup dry white wine

2 tablespoons canned tomato puree

2½ cups crushed canned tomatoes

½ pound uncooked large shrimp, peeled and deveined

1 tablespoon unsalted butter (optional)

Sea salt to taste

4 to 6 teaspoons Fresh Basil Pesto (recipe below)

Freshly grated Pecorino Romano or Parmigiano-Reggiano cheese (optional)

1. Heat a medium-size saucepot on medium and add 1 tablespoon of the olive oil. Add the onion, fennel seeds, and oregano and cook for 2 minutes with the lid on. Take the lid off and cook for another 6 minutes, stirring frequently.

2. Add the garlic and cook for another 2 minutes. Add the calamari and sauté for 3 minutes. Add the salmon and sauté for another 3 minutes. Pour in the wine and reduce by half; this will take approximately 6 minutes.

3. Add the tomato puree and crushed tomatoes, cover with a lid, and simmer the stew for 20 minutes to let the flavors meld together. Add the shrimp and cook for another 10 minutes.

4. Turn off the heat, add the butter if using, and season with salt. Cover the pot and let the stew sit for 5 minutes before serving.

5. Top each serving with 1 teaspoon of basil pesto (recipe page 95) and the grated cheese of your choice. Serve the fish sticks hot with tartar sauce and lemon wedges.

TIP

For added tenderness, you can soak the calamari in milk for 2 to 6 hours before you cook it.

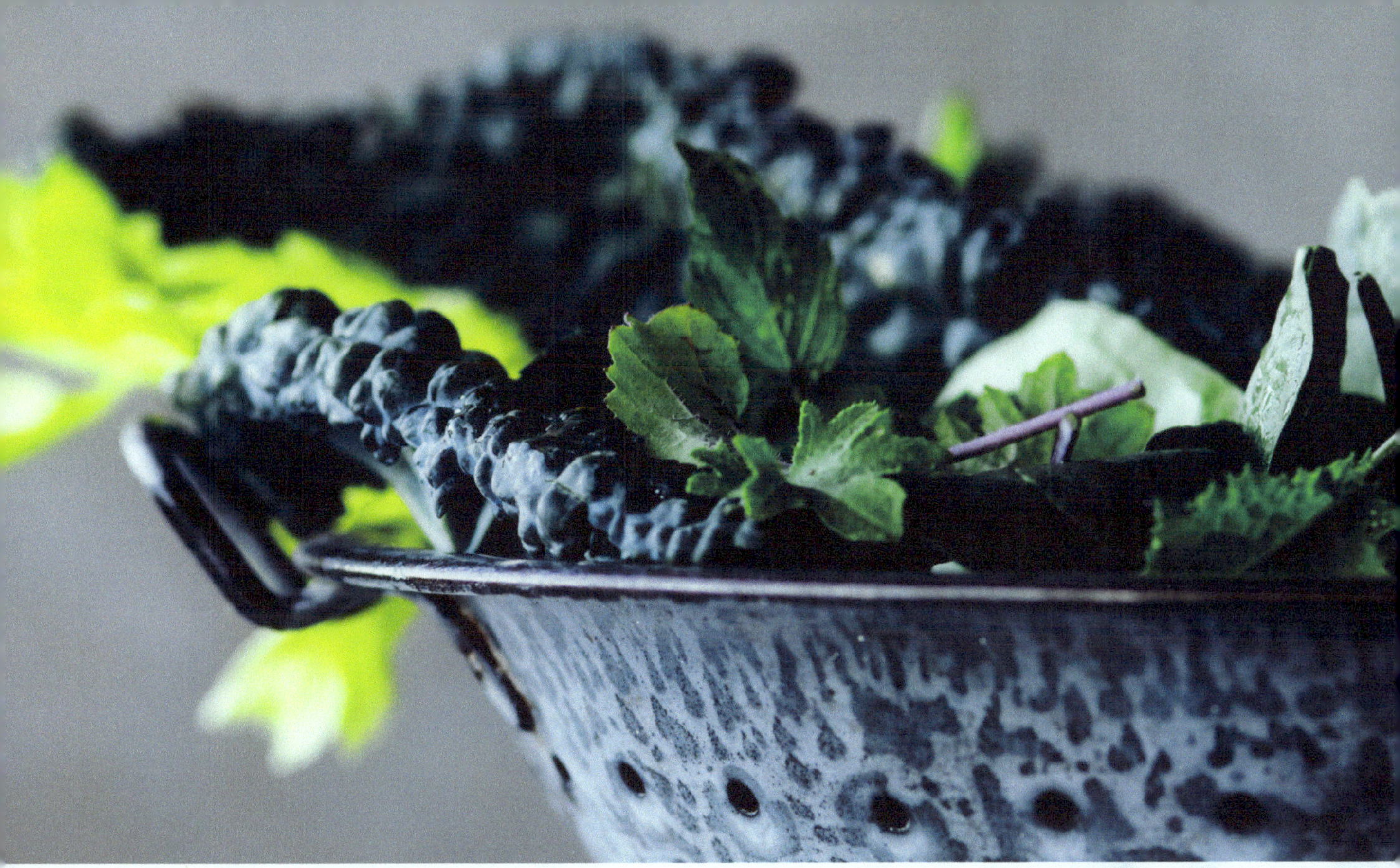

FRESH BASIL PESTO

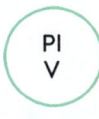

This pesto brightens up most any dish. Include a dollop on pastas, toast, meats, soups, roasted vegetables, or on our Baked Spaghetti Squash (page 118). This is a summertime go-to that tastes best when using fresh picked home-grown basil.

Makes about 1 cup

2 cups packed fresh basil leaves

⅓ cup pine nuts, lightly toasted in a dry pan

1 to 2 cloves garlic, minced

Sea salt to taste

½ cup freshly grated Pecorino Romano cheese

½ cup extra-virgin olive oil

1. Put the basil leaves, toasted pine nuts, and garlic in the bowl of a food processor and pulse for 30 seconds. Add a pinch of salt. Add the Pecorino and process for 30 seconds more, scraping down the sides of the bowls as needed. With the food processor running, slowly drizzle in the olive oil and then season with salt.

2. Serve immediately or store for up to 3 days in a tightly covered glass container.

TIP

We love using basil pesto as a salad dressing, especially with roasted veggies. To make pesto into a vinaigrette, whisk in olive oil and a touch of balsamic vinegar until the pesto is thinned and you have the flavor you want..

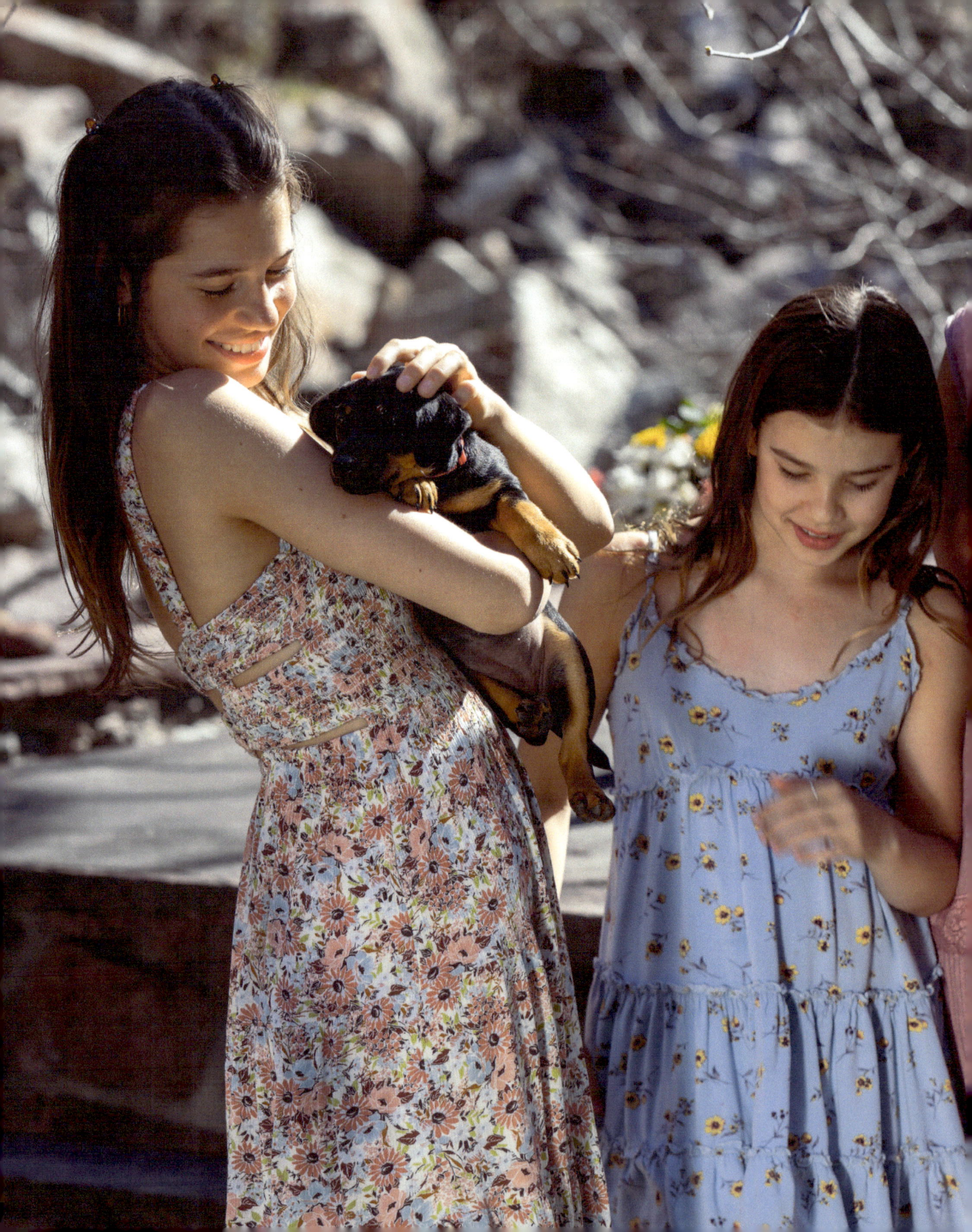

CHICKEN FINGERS

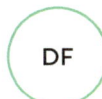

DF

Serves 4 kids or 2 adults

1 pound boneless free-range chicken thighs or breasts

2 large eggs

Sea salt to taste

1½ cups Gluten-Free Breadcrumbs (page 91)

1 teaspoon garlic powder

1 teaspoon onion powder

3 tablespoons coconut oil or extra-virgin olive oil

Dairy-Free Ranch Dressing (page 74), for serving

1. Prepare your ingredients and arrange them in the following sequence near your stovetop: Lightly pound the chicken thighs and cut them into approximately 2-inch-wide strips. In a shallow dish, lightly beat the eggs with a dash of salt. In another shallow dish, stir together the breadcrumbs, garlic powder, onion powder, and a dash of salt.

2. Dip the chicken strips into the eggs, allowing the excess to drain off, and then dip them into the breading, making sure to coat them thoroughly. Set aside on a large plate.

3. Heat 1½ tablespoons of the coconut oil in a large sauté pan or griddle on medium heat.

4. Add half of the chicken strips to the pan and cook, flipping them at least once, until they are golden brown on both sides and cooked through, about 15 minutes total. Transfer to a plate layered with paper towels to drain.

5. After the first batch is done, wipe the pan with a paper towel. Reheat the pan on medium with the remaining coconut oil and cook the rest of the chicken strips.

6. Serve with a side of our ranch dressing for dipping.

TIP

For an egg-free version, substitute 3 tablespoons canned full-fat coconut milk and 1 tablespoon olive oil per egg.

DAIRY-FREE FRIED CHICKEN

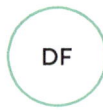

DF

Serves 4 to 6

6 cups filtered water

½ cup salt

3 to 4 pounds bone-in chicken pieces

1 (14-ounce) can full-fat coconut milk

½ tablespoon apple cider vinegar

2 cups brown rice flour

⅔ cup potato or tapioca starch

1 teaspoon sea salt, plus more for seasoning the chicken

2 teaspoons garlic powder

2 teaspoons paprika

2 teaspoons cayenne pepper

½ cup coconut oil

½ cup extra-virgin olive oil

1. In a large bowl, combine the water and salt, stirring until the salt dissolves. Add the chicken pieces to the brine and refrigerate for 2 to 8 hours. (We usually put chicken in to brine in the morning before work begins.)

2. When you're ready to fry the chicken, preheat the oven to 350°F. Drain the chicken and thoroughly pat it dry with paper towels.

3. In a mixing bowl, whisk together the coconut milk and vinegar. In another mixing bowl, mix together the flour, starch, salt, garlic powder, paprika, and cayenne.

4. Working with one piece at a time, dip the chicken into the canned coconut milk and let the excess drip off as well as you can. Dip the chicken into the flour mixture (you can double-dip for a thicker breading). Set the prepared pieces aside on a large plate.

5. Heat a large sauté pan to medium. Add ¼ cup of each of the oils, heat until lightly bubbling, and add 3 to 4 pieces of chicken to the pan. Fry the chicken on each side for 6 minutes or until deep golden brown. Drain on paper towels.

6. Working in 2 to 4 batches total, fry the rest of the chicken, making sure to strain or wipe out any burnt or crusty bits in between batches and to add more of the oil when needed.

7. When all of the chicken has been fried and drained, put it into a large baking dish and bake for approximately 25 minutes, until it reaches an internal temperature of 165°F on a meat thermometer.

8. Let sit for 5 minutes and serve. We enjoy this with our buttermilk biscuits on the side.

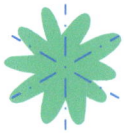

TIP

After a lot of experimentation, we chose to first fry and then bake this chicken to get the full flavor and crispy effect without fully submerging the chicken in oil. Not only does this method deliver the best taste and texture, it also makes less of a mess in the kitchen. This can also be prepared with buttermilk instead of the coconut milk and vinegar mixture, if you prefer.

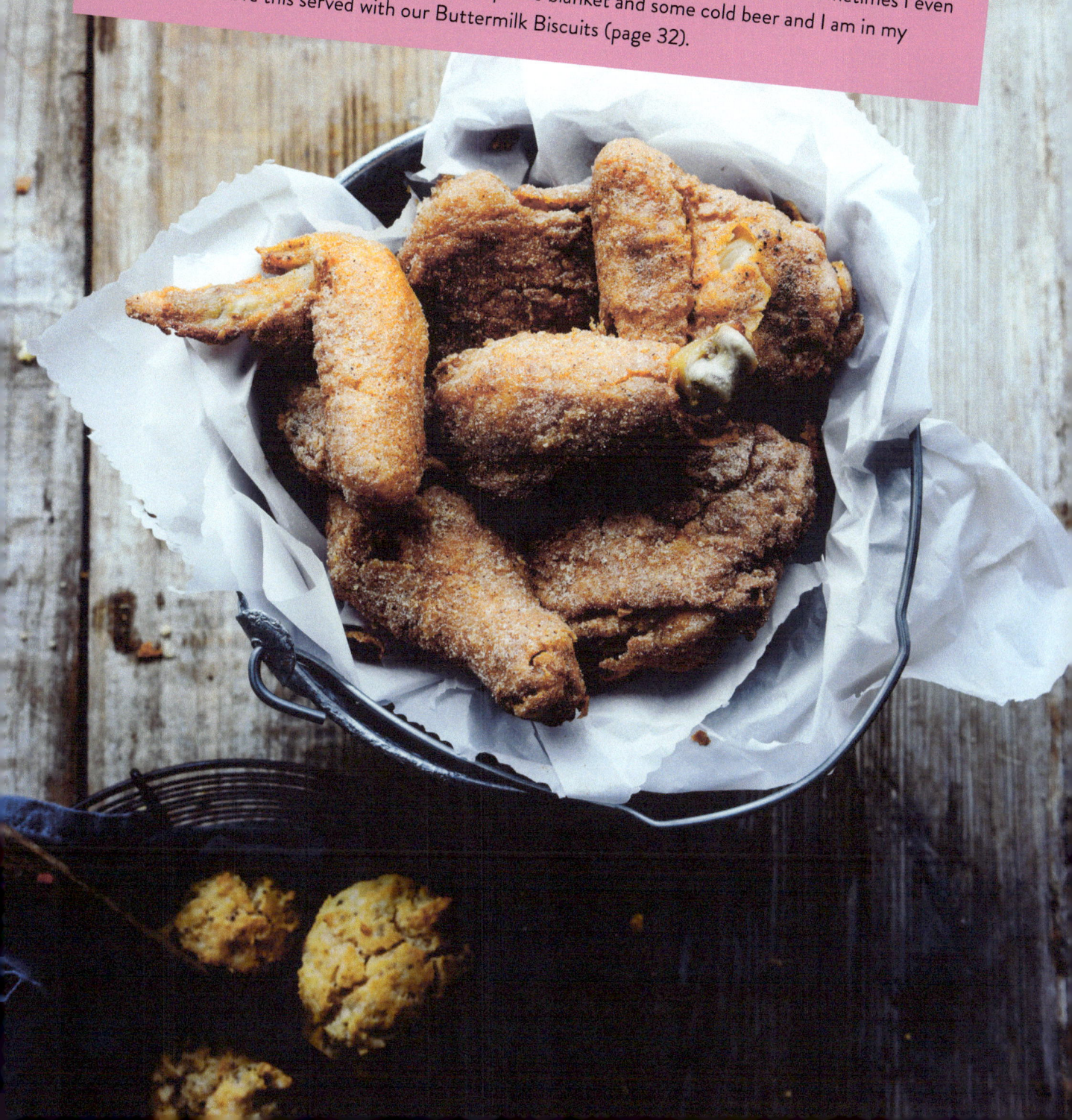

Jill: Who doesn't love fried chicken? I myself have always been a devotee (and admit that I even enjoyed buckets of it in the past). But as my diet changed, I thought those days were gone. Well, this dairy-free version, fried in a combination of coconut and olive oil, is fantastic—sometimes I even throw it in a bucket for old times' sake. Add a picnic blanket and some cold beer and I am in my happy place. I love this served with our Buttermilk Biscuits (page 32).

WHOLE ROASTED CHICKEN WITH MAPLE-ROASTED VEGETABLES

DF

This is a recipe that we hope will become one of your family favorites. The house smells so delicious, and it is a dish that is easy to love by the whole family. The sweet fruit and vegetables contrast nicely with the savory chicken.

Serves 4 to 6

2 tablespoons extra-virgin olive oil or softened unsalted butter (optional)

Sea salt

1 (4-pound) free-range roasting chicken (see Tip)

2 lemons, halved

3 cloves garlic

5 rosemary sprigs

2 tablespoons raw apple cider vinegar

1½ cups chicken stock (to make your own, see page 56)

1½ tablespoons maple syrup

1 tablespoon unsalted butter (optional)

3 apples (we like Honeycrisp or Fuji), peeled, cored, and cut into cubes

3 carrots, peeled and cut into large dice

1 large sweet potato, peeled and cut into large dice

½ onion, sliced

½ bulb fennel, sliced

1. Preheat the oven to 400°F.

2. Rub the olive oil and a generous amount of salt on the chicken. Put the lemon, garlic, and rosemary into the cavity of the chicken and set aside.

3. In a small saucepan, combine the vinegar, stock, maple syrup, butter, if using, and a healthy pinch of salt. Cook over medium heat until reduced by half.

4. In the bottom of a roasting pan or Dutch oven, arrange the apples, carrots, sweet potato, onion, and fennel to form a bed for the chicken. Pour the chicken stock mixture over the vegetables and lightly toss. Place the prepared chicken on top of the vegetables.

5. Roast the chicken for 1½ to 2 hours, until it reaches an internal temperature of 165°F on a meat thermometer.

6. Transfer the chicken to a platter and let it rest for 15 minutes. Carve the chicken and serve it over the maple-roasted vegetables.

TIP

To calculate the roasting time for a larger or smaller bird, estimate 22 to 25 minutes per pound. Even after a free-range chicken is roasted, the bones can be used to make stock. Just follow our chicken stock recipe on page 56; the only difference is you may want to simmer the bones for a couple of hours longer in order to pull out all of the nutrients and flavor.

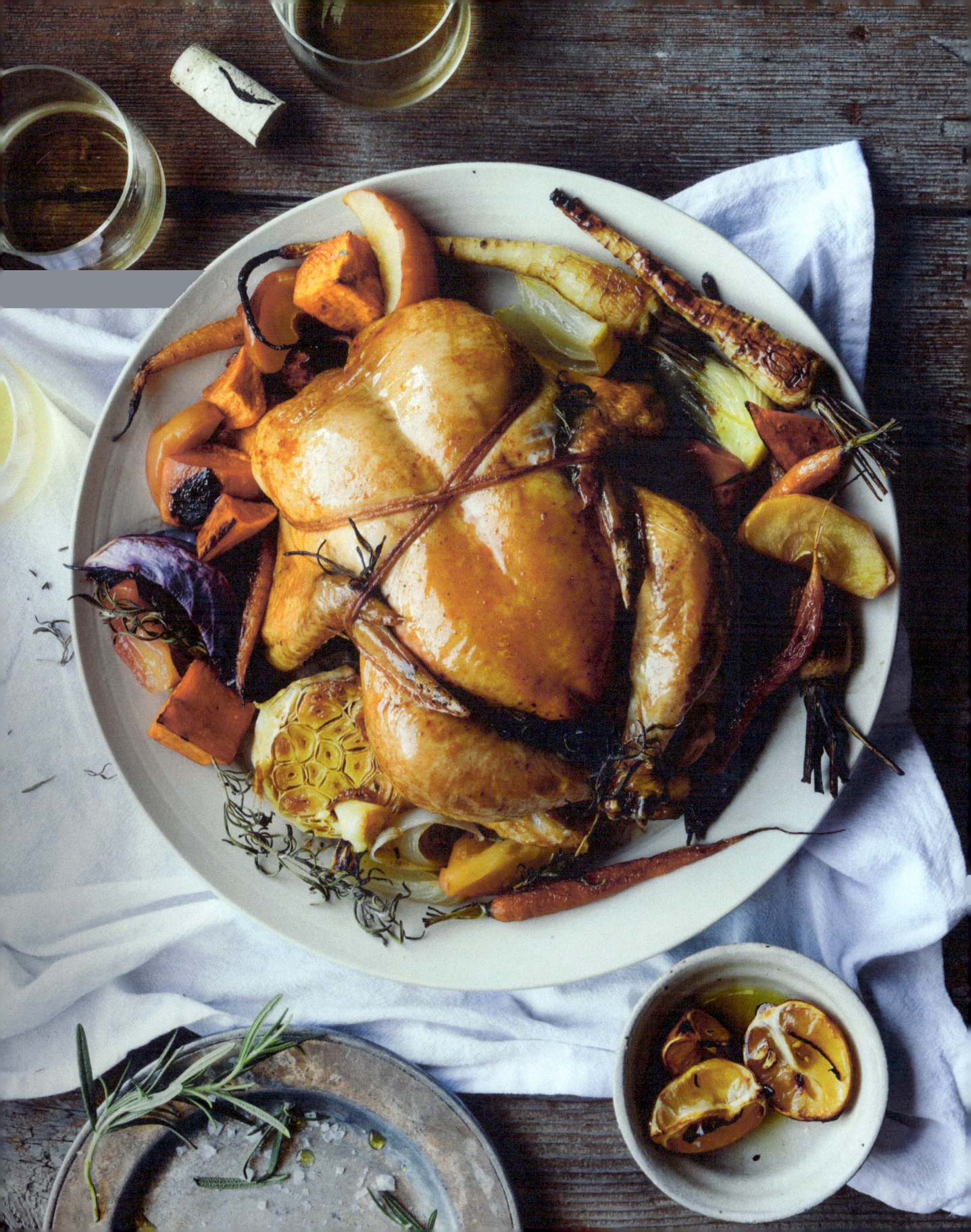

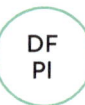

DF
PI

BARB-ECK-QUE CHICKEN

Serves 4 to 6

8 to 10 bone-in, skin-on free-range chicken thighs

¼ cup extra-virgin olive oil

¼ cup Eck's Dry Rub (recipe below)

1 cup Barbeque Sauce (recipe below)

1. Preheat an outdoor gas or charcoal grill to low heat. Scrape the hot grill plates clean with a wire brush so the chicken will cook without sticking.

2. Brush the chicken thighs lightly with the olive oil. Sprinkle the dry rub very liberally all over the thighs.

3. Grill the chicken thighs, turning and brushing them liberally with the barbeque sauce every 5 minutes or so, until the skin is super crispy and the barbeque sauce is syrupy and caramelized, 40 to 45 minutes total. (Using a meat thermometer, check that the internal temperature of the chicken has reached 165°F before removing the chicken from the grill; see Tip.)

4. Let the chicken sit for 5 minutes before serving.

TIP

As Eck always says, the way to make really yummy barbeque chicken is to cook the thighs low and slow. This brings out their flavor and a super tender consistency.

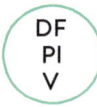

DF
PI
V

BARBEQUE SAUCE

Makes about 1 cup

1 cup canned stewed tomatoes, drained

2½ tablespoons molasses

1 tablespoon honey

2 tablespoons apple cider vinegar

¼ teaspoon dried oregano

¼ teaspoon garlic powder

¼ teaspoon ground mustard

1. Puree the stewed tomatoes in a blender.

2. Transfer the tomatoes to a saucepan, add the remaining ingredients, and simmer for 10 minutes, stirring occasionally.

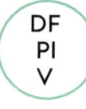

DF
PI
V

ECK'S DRY RUB

Yield: about ½ cup

¼ cup smoked paprika

1 tablespoon garlic powder

2 teaspoons sea salt

1 teaspoon cumin

1 teaspoon cayenne pepper

¼ teaspoon dry mustard

Combine all ingredients in a bowl. Store in a tightly sealed glass jar.

Jennifer: This was the dish my husband, Eric (Eck) made when my whole family came over for the first time after we were married. Coming from a big Italian family, I am very used to big meals and chaos. Eck put so much love and time into this dish that my family was hooked not only on the chicken but on my hubby as well. To this day, you'll find him standing over the grill in the summertime when the whole family gets together at our place. He is very proud of this dish and was over the moon about having it included in our cookbook.

SAUSAGE AND PEPPERS

Growing up in an expressive Italian family, many stories were told over sausage and peppers. It was a quick and easy dinner Dad would throw on the stovetop so the focus could be on family time instead of slaving over a hot stove. Serve straight out of the oven or with yummy, crusty Italian bread on the side.

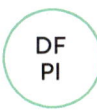

DF
PI

Serves 4 to 6

2 tablespoons extra-virgin olive oil

8 Italian-style sausages

1 large onion, sliced

sea salt to taste

2 large red bell peppers, seeded and sliced

1 cup sliced mushrooms

2 cloves garlic, minced

1. Preheat the oven to 325°F.

2. Heat a large sauté pan on medium heat for 2 minutes and then add the olive oil.

3. Add the sausages and cook, turning frequently then covering the pan to avoid splatter, until the sausages are browned on all sides, approximately 10 minutes. Put aside on a plate.

4. To the same pan, add the onion and a pinch of salt and cook for about 4 minutes, until translucent. Add the peppers and mushrooms and sauté until soft, approximately 8 minutes. Add the garlic and sauté for about 2 minutes more, stirring occasionally.

5. Transfer the mixed vegetables to a large baking pan (15 x 11 inches is ideal) and top with the sausages. Bake for approximately 30 minutes to allow all of the flavors and juices to mingle. Serve straight out of the oven.

TIP

Sausage and peppers make great leftovers. Try them on sandwiches or over pasta.

SEARED PORK CHOPS WITH BRAISED CABBAGE AND FENNEL

DF
PI

Serves 4 to 6

Sea salt

4 to 6 bone-in shoulder-blade chops or center-cut bone-in chops, about 6 ounces each (see Tip)

2 tablespoons extra-virgin olive oil, if needed

¼ onion, thinly sliced

½ teaspoon caraway seeds

½ large fennel bulb or 1 small bulb, cored and thinly sliced

½ large cabbage, cored and thinly sliced

2 cups chicken stock (to make your own, see page 56)

10 sprigs fresh dill

3 to 4 slices bacon (optional)

1. Preheat the oven to 300°F.

2. Generously salt the pork chops on both sides.

3. Heat the olive oil in a Dutch oven or heavy-bottomed pot to medium-high. Sear the chops on both sides until browned, approximately 4 minutes per side. Set the chops aside on a large plate, leaving the fat in the pan.

4. If more oil is needed, add the olive oil to the pot, then add the onion and caraway seeds and sauté until the onion is soft and translucent. Add the fennel and sauté until soft, and then add the cabbage and sauté until soft. Season the cabbage mixture with salt.

5. Pour in the stock and return the pork to the pot. Top each pork chop with dill sprigs and bacon strips, if using. Cover and braise for 1½ hours, until tender.

6. Chop the bacon. Remove and discard the dill sprigs. Serve the pork and cabbage immediately.

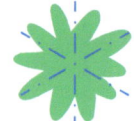

TIP

There are many cuts of pork you could use for this dish, however, we recommend bone-in because it has the best flavor and adds flavor to the cabbage and broth as well. We like to serve this with Apple Pear Puree (page 124) on the side.

Jessica: My husband is Czech. He loves anything pork, schnitzeled, or served with beer. This is for him.

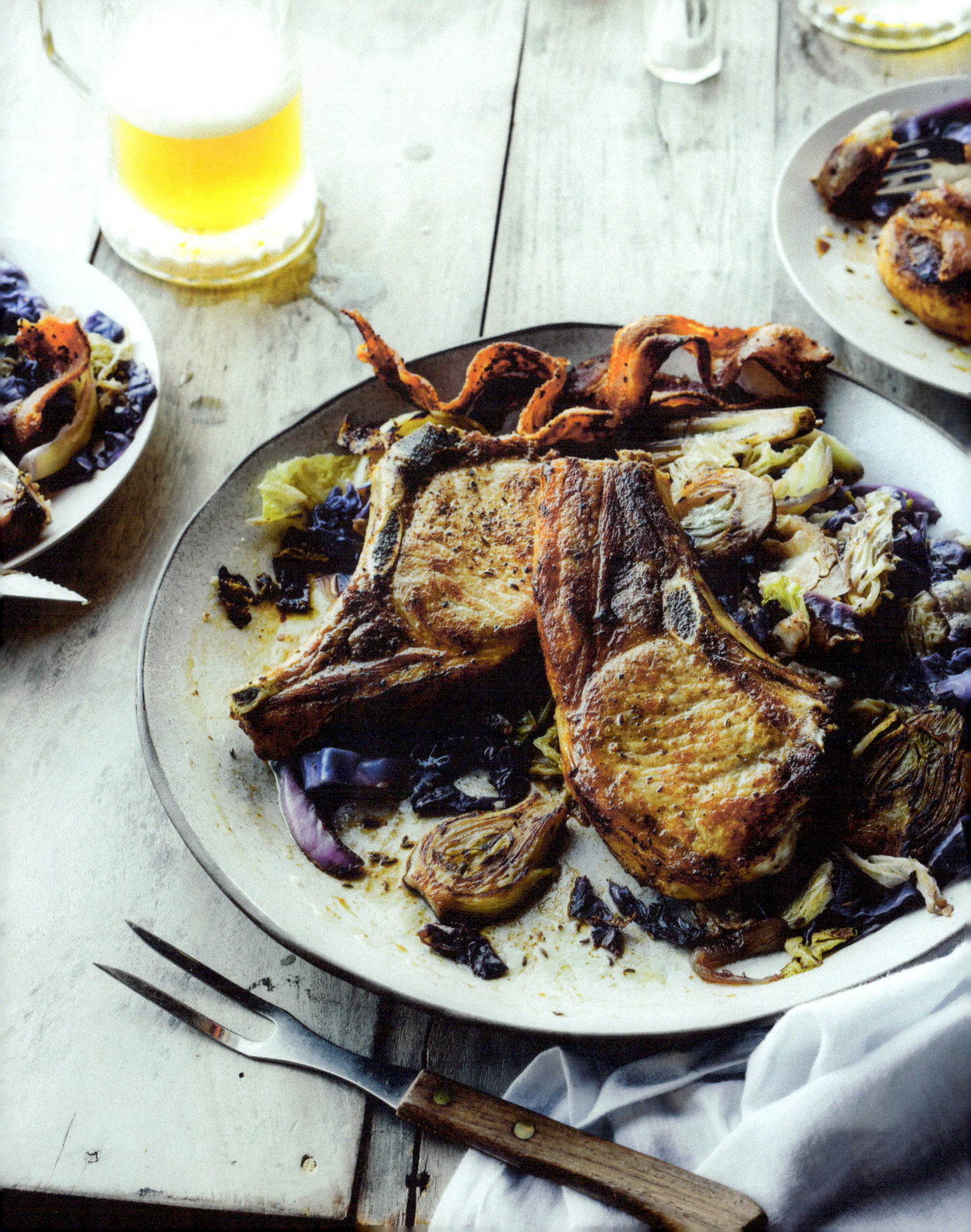

BEAN-FREE CHILI

DF
PI

Serves 4 to 6

Sea salt

2 tablespoons extra-virgin olive oil

½ small onion, medium diced

2 green bell peppers, seeded and medium diced

1 poblano pepper, medium diced

1 yellow squash, medium diced

½ cup sliced mushrooms

2 cloves garlic, minced

2½ pounds grass-fed ground beef

¼ cup chili powder

1 tablespoon ground cumin

1 cup chicken stock (to make your own, see page 56)

3½ cups canned diced tomatoes (two 14-ounce cans)

3 tablespoons chopped cilantro, for serving (optional)

sour cream, for serving (optional)

Fresh lime wedges

Sea salt to taste

1. Heat a large, heavy-bottomed pot to medium and add 1 tablespoon of the olive oil.

2. Add the onions and sauté for 4 minutes. Add the green peppers and poblano; sauté for 4 minutes. Add the remaining 1 tablespoon olive oil along with the squash, mushrooms, and garlic; sauté for 4 minutes. Add the beef, chili powder, and cumin; sauté for 4 minutes. Stir in the chicken stock and diced tomatoes, cover the pot, and simmer on low for 45 minutes, until flavors are melded. Add sea salt to taste.

3. Garnish with cilantro, sour cream, and lime wedges and serve.

TIP

You can get very creative with the vegetables as long as you keep the peppers called for in this recipe. Leftovers can be frozen in an airtight container for up to 2 months.

Jessica: This is a quick, easy recipe that is very satisfying on cold fall and winter nights. Both of my kids eat it voraciously, which makes me happy because it is a quick preparation and an easy cleanup!

GRASS-FED BEEF STEW

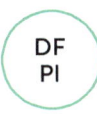

DF
PI

This is a nourishing, hearty dish that is extremely warming during the winter months. We enjoy it as an après ski meal in front of a fire to replenish energy and to warm our bones. This stew is also a hit for casual entertaining and easily scales up for big-batch cooking.

Serves 4 to 6

2 tablespoons extra-virgin olive oil or coconut oil

1 small yellow onion, chopped

Sea salt to taste

1 ½ pounds grass-fed beef or buffalo roast, cut into 1-inch cubes

2 tablespoons gluten-free Worcestershire sauce

¾ cup sliced mushrooms

1 or 2 cloves garlic, minced

½ cup sherry or red wine

1½ teaspoons ground nutmeg

1 teaspoon fennel seeds

3 to 4 thyme sprigs

2 rosemary sprigs

5 cups beef or chicken stock (to make your own, see page 55 or 56)

2 small carrots, peeled and diced

2 celery stalks, peeled and diced

1 small sweet potato, peeled and diced

2 tablespoons tapioca or arrowroot flour

1 tablespoon unsalted butter, optional

1. Heat a heavy casserole pot over medium to high heat and add the oil and onion. Cook until soft, approximately 5 minutes. Season with salt. Add the beef and cook for approximately 5 minutes, until browned.

2. Add the Worcestershire sauce and mushrooms and cook for 5 minutes until mushrooms are cooked through. Then add garlic and cook for 2 minutes, stirring occasionally.

3. Add the sherry and reduce the liquid by half, then add the nutmeg, fennel seeds, thyme, rosemary, and the stock. Bring to a boil.

4. Add the carrots, celery, and sweet potato, reduce the heat to a simmer, and cook with the lid on for 15 minutes, until the vegetables are tender. Remove the lid and cook on medium heat for another 15 minutes (this will start the evaporation and thickening process).

5. Add the flour to a measuring cup or bowl. Mix in a few tablespoons of the beef broth until the flour is completely dissolved. Add the flour slurry to the pot and cook on medium-low heat for approximately 1½ hours, until the flavors are melded.

6. Turn off the heat. Stir in the butter if you are using it and let the stew sit for 10 minutes with the lid on.

7. Divide among bowls and serve immediately. Leftovers can be stored in an airtight container in the refrigerator for up to 5 days.

TIP

We like to serve this stew over Cauliflower Mashers (page 120) or on its own with crusty gluten-free bread or our Buttermilk Biscuits (page 32). You can replace the sherry or red wine with additional stock if preferred.

DAD'S POT OF SAUCE WITH MEATBALLS

Whenever we go back home to New Jersey, this is what Dad prepares on our first night. The scent of this sauce is home to us; it is hearty, healing, and nourishing and represents family, love, indulgence, and our Jersey Italian heritage. We enjoy opening a nice bottle of red wine, settling back in with our brother and parents, and catching up on each other's lives. Now watching the kids devour the sauce and meatballs feels full circle. Home really is where the heart is. Thanks for this one, Dad.

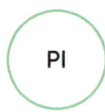

PI

Serves 4 to 6

2 tablespoons extra-virgin olive oil

1 medium onion, chopped

1 red bell pepper, seeded and chopped

3 cloves garlic, minced

1 (28-ounce) can diced tomatoes

1 (16-ounce) can crushed tomatoes

2 teaspoons dried oregano

Sea salt to taste

1 cup sliced cremini mushrooms

2 tablespoons tomato paste

2 tablespoons chopped fresh basil

1. Heat a large saucepan to medium-high and add the olive oil. Add the onion and pepper, lower the heat to medium, and sauté for 8 minutes, until the onion begins to turn translucent. Add the garlic and cook for 2 to 3 minutes more, stirring frequently.

2. Stir in the diced and crushed tomatoes, the oregano, and salt. Let simmer for approximately 15 minutes.

3. Add the mushrooms and the tomato paste to the pot. Cover and cook for another 30 to 45 minutes, stirring occasionally.

4. Add the meatballs, cover the pot, and continue to cook for another 30 minutes. Add the fresh basil 10 minutes before you plan on serving the sauce. Divide among bowls and serve immediately. Leftovers can be stored in an airtight container in the refrigerator for up to 5 days.

TIP

Both the sauce and the meatballs can be made in bigger batches and kept frozen. You can freeze the meatballs right along with the sauce and heat them back up together in a pot over medium heat.

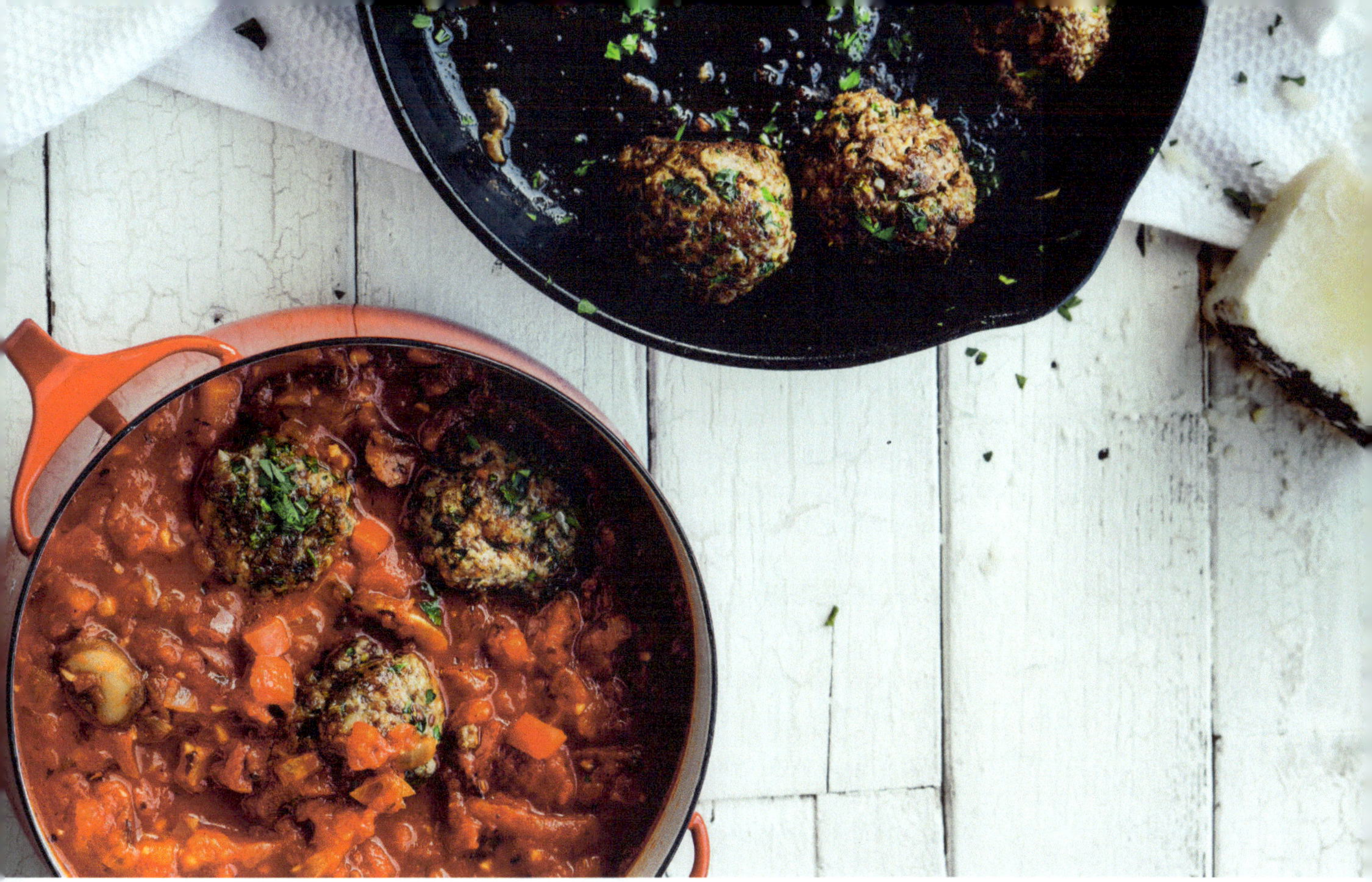

DAD'S MEATBALLS

PI

*Makes approximately
10 meatballs*

1 pound grass-fed ground
beef (we prefer 85%
lean for juiciness)

2 cloves garlic, minced

⅓ cup fresh parsley,
chopped

⅓ cup grated Pecorino
Romano cheese

⅓ cup ground flax seeds

1 large egg

1 teaspoon sea salt

2 to 3 tablespoons
extra-virgin olive oil

1. In a large mixing bowl, combine the beef, garlic, parsley, Romano, flax, egg, and salt, using your hands to mix all the ingredients together.

2. Form the ground beef mixture into approximately 10 meatballs, allowing about 2 heaping tablespoons for each.

3. Heat a large sauté pan to medium-high. Add the olive oil. Sauté the meatballs on all sides to brown them evenly, about 8-10 minutes total.

4. Add the meatballs to pot of sauce and cook for another 30 minutes, as described in step 4 of recipe above (see Tip).

TIP

The meatballs will still be undercooked when you add them to the sauce. They will finish cooking in the sauce. If you are making them without the sauce, finish by baking the meatballs in a preheated 375°F oven for another 15 minutes.

BRAISED SHORT RIBS

When we think of nourishing comfort food, this is one of the first recipes that comes to mind. We found that adding port contributes a hint of sweetness to the earthy flavor. (The alcohol cooks off during the cooking.) This is a surefire crowd pleaser for parties or big family gatherings and is especially delicious served with our Cauliflower Mashers (page 120).

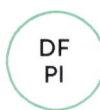

DF
Pl

Serves 4 to 6

2 tablespoons extra-virgin olive oil

5 pounds bone-in grass-fed short ribs

Sea salt to taste

2 carrots, chopped

2 stalks celery, diced

1 onion, chopped

2½ cups red wine

1½ cups port wine

5 cups beef or chicken stock (to make your own, see page 55 or 56), plus more if needed

4 thyme sprigs

4 rosemary sprigs

2 cloves garlic, minced

1 tablespoon unsalted butter (optional)

1. Preheat the oven to 325°F.

2. In a large Dutch oven, heat the olive oil on high until shimmering. Season the short ribs with a generous amount of salt. Add the short ribs to the hot pan and sear until all sides are deeply caramelized. Set aside on a platter.

3. Add the carrots, celery, and onion to the pan juices in the Dutch oven along with a dash of salt. Sauté on medium heat until the vegetables are caramelized and golden brown. Transfer the vegetables to the same platter as the short ribs.

4. Deglaze the pot with half of the wine and half of the port and reduce the liquid by half.

5. Return the short ribs and cooked vegetables to the Dutch oven. Add the stock, thyme and rosemary, and the garlic. The liquid should cover most of the ribs. If not, add more stock or water. Cover the pot with a lid and bake in the oven for 2½ hours, until the ribs are tender.

6. Remove the pot from the oven and transfer the ribs to a platter to rest. Strain the cooking liquid into a pot and reduce by half over medium heat to thicken into a sauce consistency.

7. Remove the sauce from the heat. Stir in butter if using and season with sea salt if necessary. Serve the short ribs with the sauce poured over it.

TIP

This recipe can also be made with bone-in lamb, pork. or buffalo. If you choose to prepare this recipe without wine or port, you can use additional stock instead.

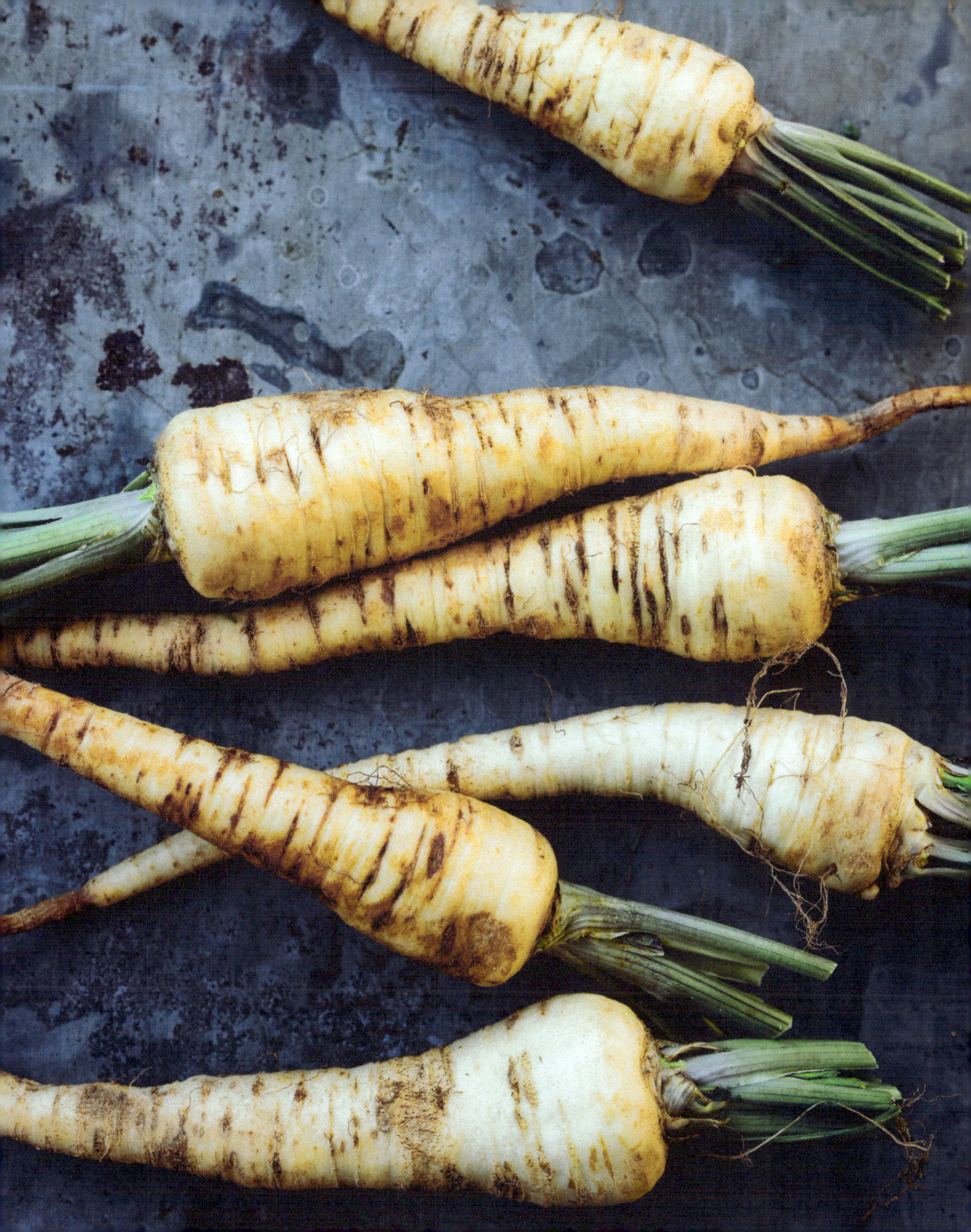

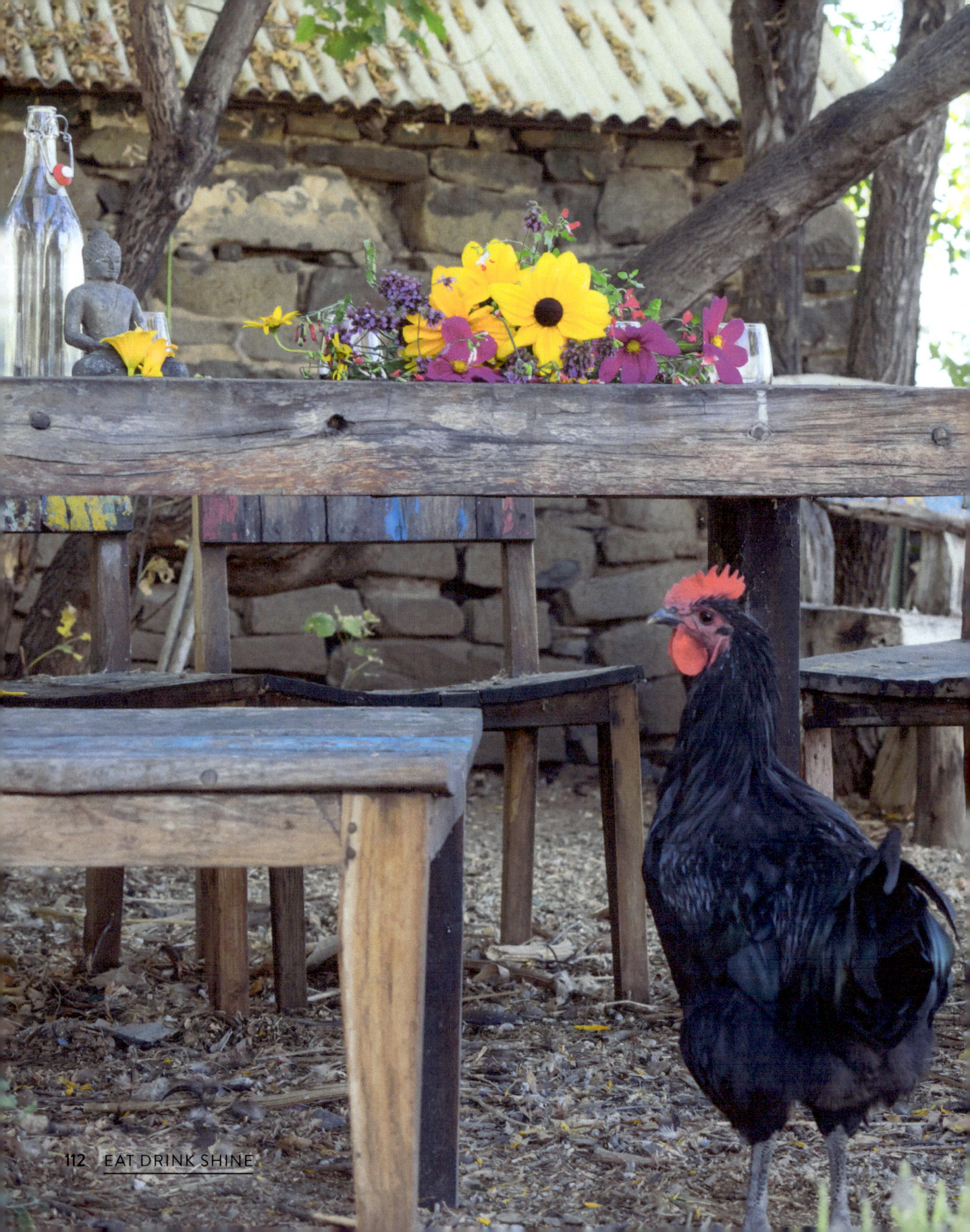

WHERE DID YOU COME FROM? THE IMPORTANCE OF SOURCING YOUR FOOD.

For us humans, where a person comes from, what their upbringing was like, and how they were raised strongly influences how they view the world and how they interact with other people and with their environment. It is the same for fruits, veggies, and meats: Where they come from and how they were grown dictates how they taste and, just as importantly, what they are made of, that is, their nutritional content. As we have mentioned before, your food literally becomes you. It is broken down in your body, enters through your cell walls, and fuels every part of you. So, don't you want to know where your food comes from and how it was grown?

An apple often is not just an apple, as it can have up to 30 pesticides lurking on its skin and within its flesh. Whatever is on and in the food is also ingested by you. If there are pesticides on your vegetables, even if you scrub them, only some of the chemicals are removed. Pesticides can poison our insides, not to mention pollute our outside environment, including water sources and the air we breathe. These poisons have been proven to cause many different illnesses. We may not be able to control the air we breathe, but we can control what food we decide to put into our bodies.

Many factory-farmed meats contain antibiotics and hormones. Antibiotics are given to animals living in unsanitary, cramped conditions to combat disease, and hormones are given to make them grow faster and to increase milk production in cattle. Not only is this inhumane for the animals, but we are also ingesting these hormones and antibiotics as we eat

the meat and drink the milk. The same goes with most farmed fish, where pesticides and antibiotics are often sprayed on the fish to kill bacteria, disease, and parasites before the fish reaches the store. It pollutes our oceans and harms marine life. Not sounding too appetizing now, is it?

We highly recommend using local and organic ingredients whenever possible. Not only do these foods have the highest amount of vitamins, minerals, and more nutritional value and flavor, but they also support your local farmers and natural grocers and help build a sustainable ecosystem for your community.

Another huge factor in healthy sourcing of ingredients is choosing grass-fed meats. Why grass fed? The way animals are fed has a big effect on the nutrient composition of the meat. In their natural settings, animals such as cows, sheep, and bison live on a healthy diet of grasses. Most of the animals raised in feedlots are started out on grass and then finished on grain. When these animals are fed grain, they are forced to eat a food that is not part of their natural diet. This causes stress on their bodies and the may be less healthy.

A grass-finished animal is higher in nutrients, especially omega-3s, which are very healthy for our bodies. Thus, eating grass-fed meat is incredibly nutritious. It is usually more expensive than its grain fed counterpart. If this is a concern, you can purchase less expensive grass-fed cuts and cook them lower and longer in stews and roasts. You may also

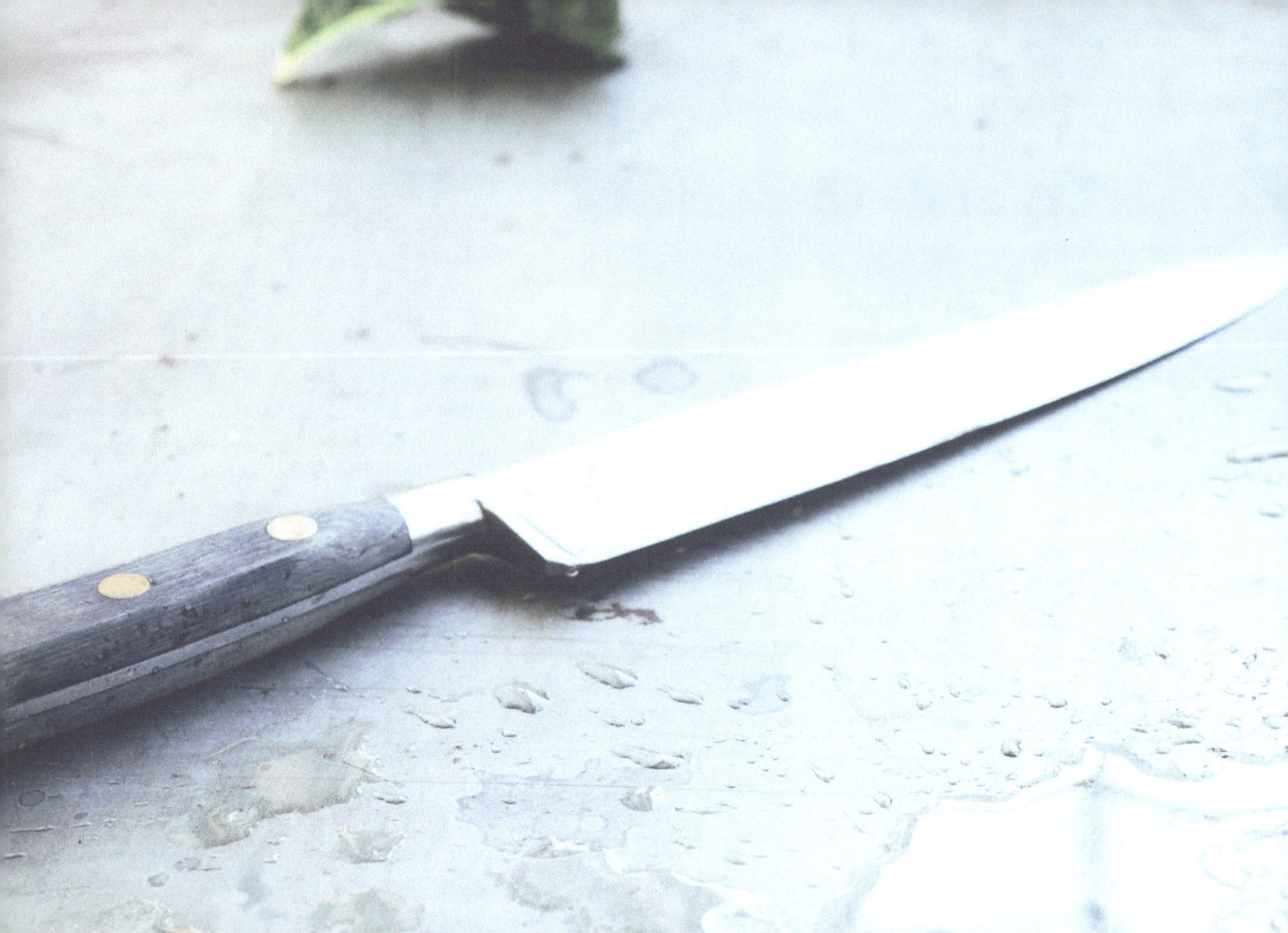

find a farm in your area that sells animals by the half or quarter, an economical way to purchase meat. There is a flavor difference, too: Grass-fed meat has a more concentrated, cleaner flavor than grain fed. It is also leaner, so when we're searing or grilling a grass-fed steak, we prefer to cook it to no more than medium-rare unless we'll be braising it afterward.

We feel it is very important to use free-range or even organic chicken if you can find it. Factory farmed, commercial birds are cooped up to where they can't move much at all, they are being fed unnatural sources of food, and not only is it inhumane but it changes the composition of the chickens and the nutritional value. Free-range are healthier birds that can wander, be in sunlight, and eat more natural forms of feed like insects and

leftover crop. Free-range, however, can also be fed the same unnatural feed as factory farmed birds but organic chickens are fed certified organic feed so it ensures the best meat possible. Free range and organic chickens are higher in omega-3 fatty acids and Vitamin A & E. They are all around healthier for them and for you. So as we talk about "you are what you eat," it is good to keep in mind that you are also ingesting what your cows, fish, and chickens are ingesting so be mindful of it as part of sourcing your animal proteins.

To understand your food and how it translates in your body is to empower yourself and truly thrive. Food is multidimensional in that it nourishes the mind, body, and heart on both a physical and emotional level.

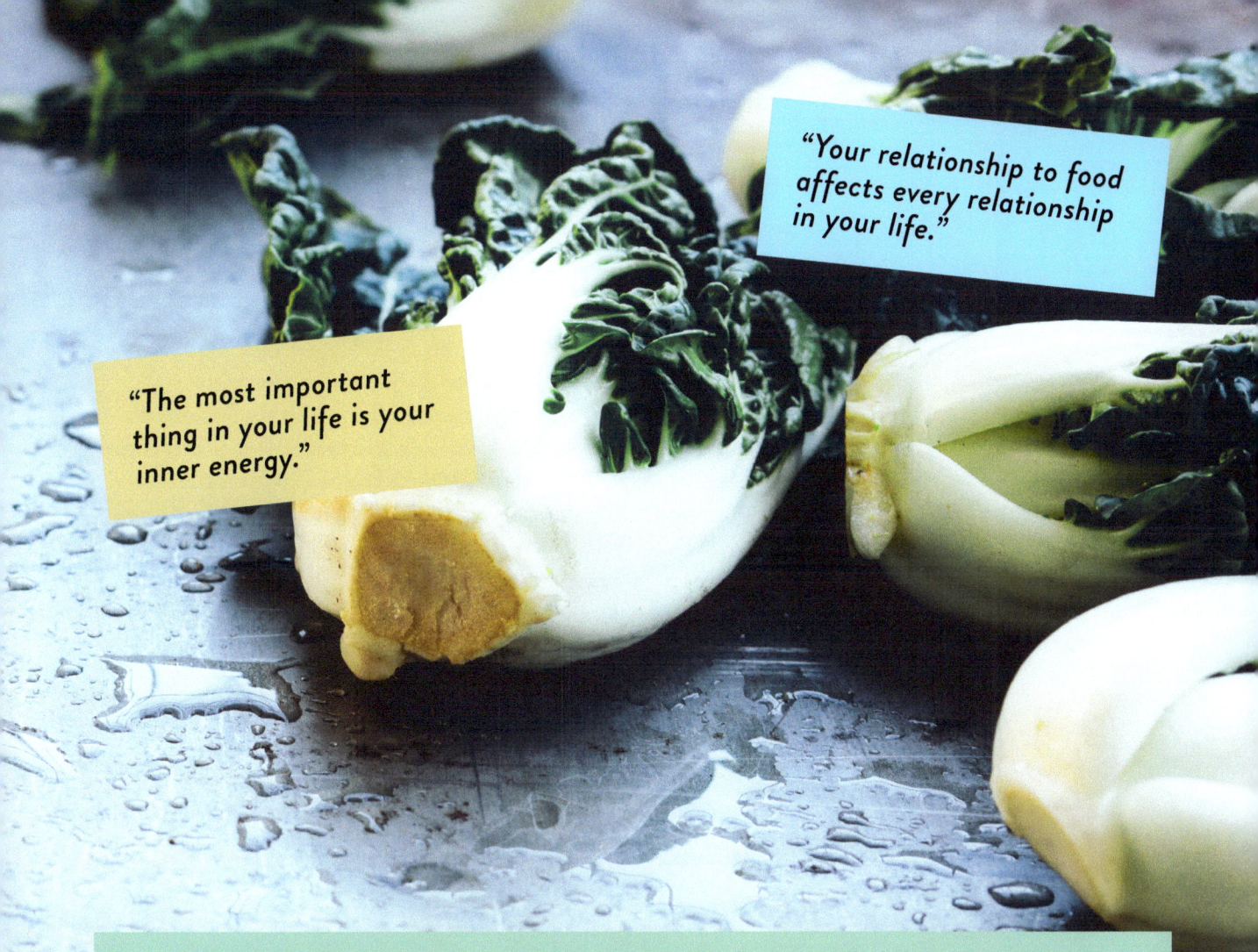

"Your relationship to food affects every relationship in your life."

"The most important thing in your life is your inner energy."

VEGGIE SIDES & MAINS

We love having snack foods on hand to munch on throughout the day that are substantial enough to keep us energized. We also have a lot of people coming into the restaurant who want to "graze," trying a little bit of everything, and the small dishes in this chapter are among their favorites. These also serve as creative components alongside our seared meats and other entrées. In keeping with a Paleo-inspired way of eating, we've included many fun "alternative" recipes that replace grains with vegetables. It keeps things nutritious and delicious!

APPLE PEAR PUREE

Apple picking as kids was a favorite way to spend the day with our many aunties, uncles, and cousins. Our mom was one of 12 kids, so we had an abundance of both. We used to pile in the station wagon with the hatchback down and scope out the best trees, then we'd pick and picnic all day long. We had apples for weeks, so we would get creative with recipes and this puree one of our favorites. We loved it as a snack or a side. For this recipe, we like to use the sweeter apples, such as Gala, Honeycrisp, or Fuji.

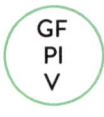

GF
PI
V

Makes about 3 cups

4 large apples, peeled, cored, and chopped into about 8 pieces

2 large pears, peeled, cored, and chopped into about 8 pieces

1 cup apple juice or water (see Tip)

2 teaspoons fresh lemon juice

1 teaspoon ground cinnamon

¼ teaspoon ground nutmeg

1 teaspoon vanilla extract (to make your own, see page 163)

1. In a heavy bottom pot over medium-low heat, combine all of the ingredients and cook for about 25 minutes, stirring occasionally. Transfer to a blender and puree until smooth.

2. Serve either warm or cold. The puree will keep in the refrigerator, stored in an airtight container, for 5 to 7 days.

TIP

The apple juice or water will only cover the bottom of the pan. It is used to steam the apple and pear; most of it will evaporate during cooking.

GRILLED BROCCOLI WITH LEMON

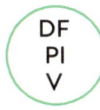

Growing up, we'd often spend the summer on the Jersey shore with our many cousins—our extended family would rent multiple houses on the same block. In the evenings, we would wheel the grills down the street to one house so we had enough grill space to cook for everybody. There was a lot of laughter and a lot of cheap beer. This broccoli was a quick and easy green addition to all of the meat and seafood. It is also a wonderful addition to salads.

Serves 4 to 6

2 heads broccoli

¼ cup extra-virgin olive oil

1½ tablespoons balsamic vinegar

3 tablespoons fresh lemon juice

Sea salt to taste

1. Preheat grill to medium or medium-high.

2. Meanwhile, prepare the broccoli by cutting off about three-quarters of the stems and cutting each head into large florets. It is important to keep these pieces large enough so that they don't quickly burn or fall through the grill grate.

3. Mix together the oil, vinegar, lemon juice, and salt in a large mixing bowl. Add the broccoli and toss to coat.

4. Transfer the broccoli to the grill, reserving the remaining dressing. Grill on all sides until the broccoli is lightly charred and softened, 10 to 15 minutes (see Tip).

5. Return the grilled broccoli to the mixing bowl and toss with the reserved dressing to coat. Chop the broccoli into smaller florets and serve.

TIP

It is okay for the broccoli to get darker, and even charred, in some places. This adds to the grilled flavor.

BAKED SPAGHETTI SQUASH

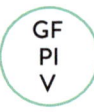

GF
PI
V

Squash is full of antioxidants, low in carbs, and results in glowing skin. This dish is a great Paleo alternative to pasta and will play well with your favorite pasta sauces.

Serves 4 to 6

1 spaghetti squash

2 tablespoons extra-virgin olive oil

Sea salt to taste

1. Preheat the oven to 425°F.

2. Cut off the stem ends of the spaghetti squash and scoop out the seeds. Drizzle each half with the olive oil and sprinkle with salt.

3. Place the squash, flesh side down, on a baking sheet, and bake for approximately 45 minutes. Let cool slightly.

4. Using a fork, scrape the spaghetti squash strands into a bowl. Serve warm as an alternative to pasta, or as a side dish with butter or more olive oil and salt.

TIP

We love sautéing wild mushrooms, garlic, tomatoes, and sage and then adding the squash for a simple and delicious fall dish.

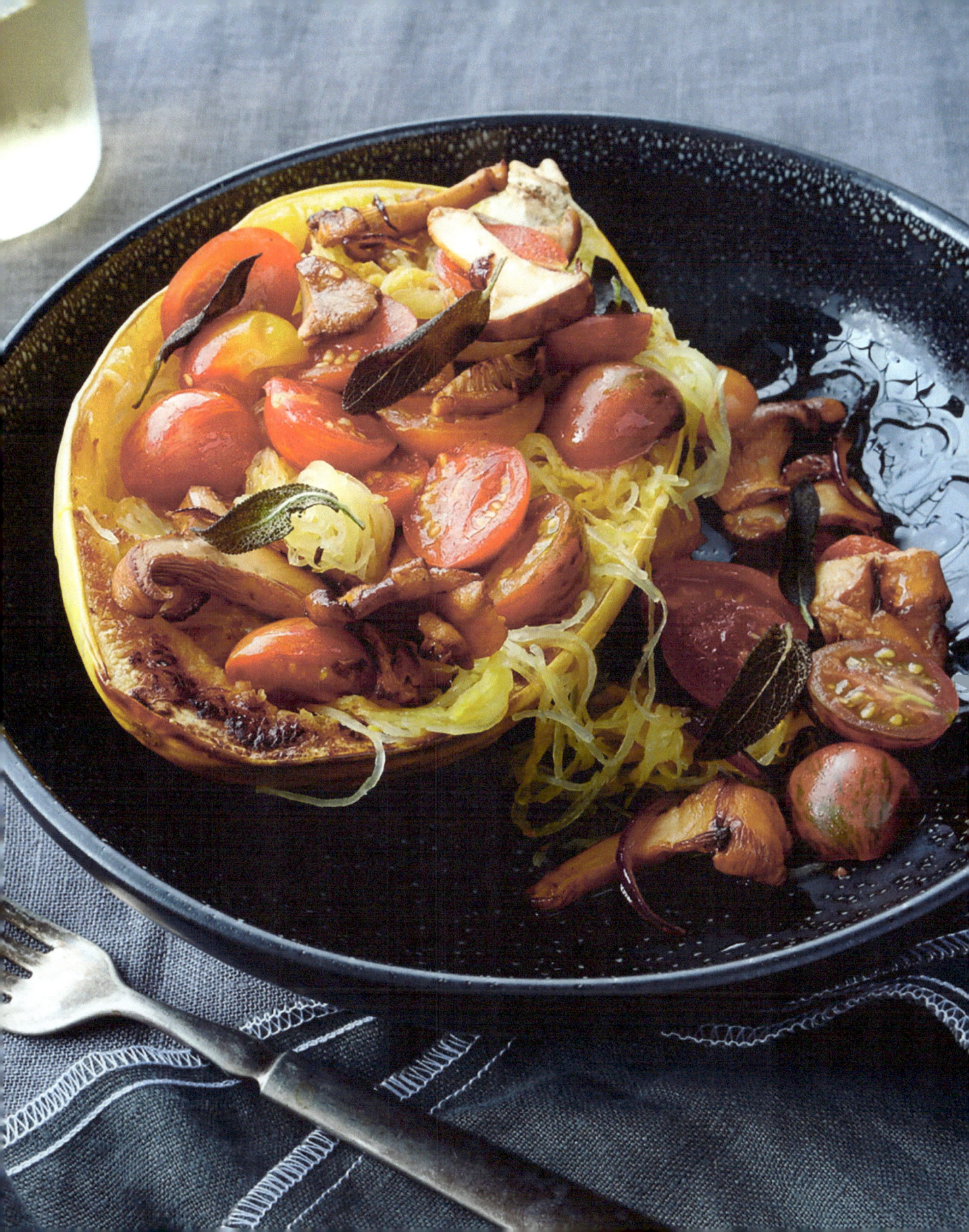

CAULIFLOWER MASHERS

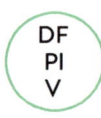

**DF
Pl
V**

A Paleo alternative to mashed potatoes, this is a Shine favorite that we serve with stews and as a side with meat or fish. If you leave out the rosemary, it makes a nourishing baby food as well.

Serves 4 to 6

1 large head cauliflower, broken into florets

1 tablespoon coconut oil

1 teaspoon chopped rosemary

2 tablespoons nutritional yeast

Sea salt to taste

1. Bring 2 cups water to a boil in a large saute pan. Add the cauliflower, cover, and steam for approximately 12 minutes. The cauliflower is done when you can pierce it with a fork.

2. Drain the cauliflower, reserving 1 cup of the cooking water (see Tip). Pour the reserved water and cauliflower into a food processor and process until smooth.

3. Add the coconut oil, rosemary, nutritional yeast, and salt and process until fully incorporated. Store in the refrigerator in an airtight container for up to 5 days.

TIP

If you like a thicker consistency, add less liquid. For additional flavor, you can substitute chicken stock for the water.

CAULIFLOWER RICE

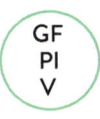

GF
PI
V

A Paleo alternative to rice, this has a very similar texture and holds juices and flavors really well. We love serving it with roasted veggies or as a side dish to any protein, with eggs, or anywhere else you would use rice.

Makes 2 cups

1 head cauliflower, outer leaves removed

1 tablespoon extra-virgin olive oil, coconut oil, or butter

Sea salt to taste

1. Using your hands, break apart the cauliflower into large florets. Chop the core into smaller pieces.

2. Working in two or three batches, process the cauliflower for 30 seconds, stopping to mix in the larger pieces. Continue for 2 to 3 minutes until the cauliflower resembles small pieces of rice. Repeat with the remaining batches. At this point, the rice can be eaten raw (see Tip), or proceed with the cooking instructions below.

3. Place a large pan over medium heat. Add the coconut oil and sauté the cauliflower rice for 10 to 12 minutes, stirring frequently, until the rice is softened and cooked through.

4. Stir in salt to taste and serve immediately, or store in the refrigerator for up to 5 days.

TIP

Add raw Cauliflower Rice to salads and soups for additional crunch.

CAULIFLOWER FRIED RICE

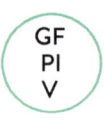

GF
PI
V

This is our cauliflower rice taken to another dimension. The additional veggies make it a satisfying vegetarian main dish. Tamari is almost always gluten-free (check the bottle!), is less salty than typical soy sauce, and can be used in place of it in any recipe.

Serves 4

2 tablespoons coconut oil or olive oil

3 large eggs, beaten

½ cup finely chopped carrots

2 tablespoons finely chopped yellow onion

½ cup chopped green beans or frozen peas

½ cup chopped mushrooms (we like to use shiitakes)

2 cups Cauliflower Rice (page 121)

¼ cup gluten-free tamari

2 tablespoons toasted sesame oil

¼ cup thinly sliced green onion

Sea salt to taste

1. In a large sauté pan over low-medium heat, heat 1 tablespoon coconut oil. Pour in the whisked eggs, swirling them slightly to get a thin, even layer on the bottom of the pan. Continue to cook over low-medium heat until just cooked through. Slide the cooked eggs onto a cutting board and chop into a small dice. Set aside.

2. Raise the heat to medium-high and add the remaining tablespoon of coconut oil to the pan. Add the carrots and sauté for 4 to 5 minutes. Add the onion, green beans, and mushrooms and sauté for 5 minutes. Add the cauliflower rice and cook for an additional 5 minutes, stirring frequently until lightly browned and cooked through. Add the tamari and mix well for 1 minute.

3. Turn off the heat and add the sesame oil, reserved cooked eggs, and green onion. Mix well, add salt to taste, and serve.

 **TIP**

Cooked ground beef or turkey can be added with the eggs and green onion to make this a hearty main dish.

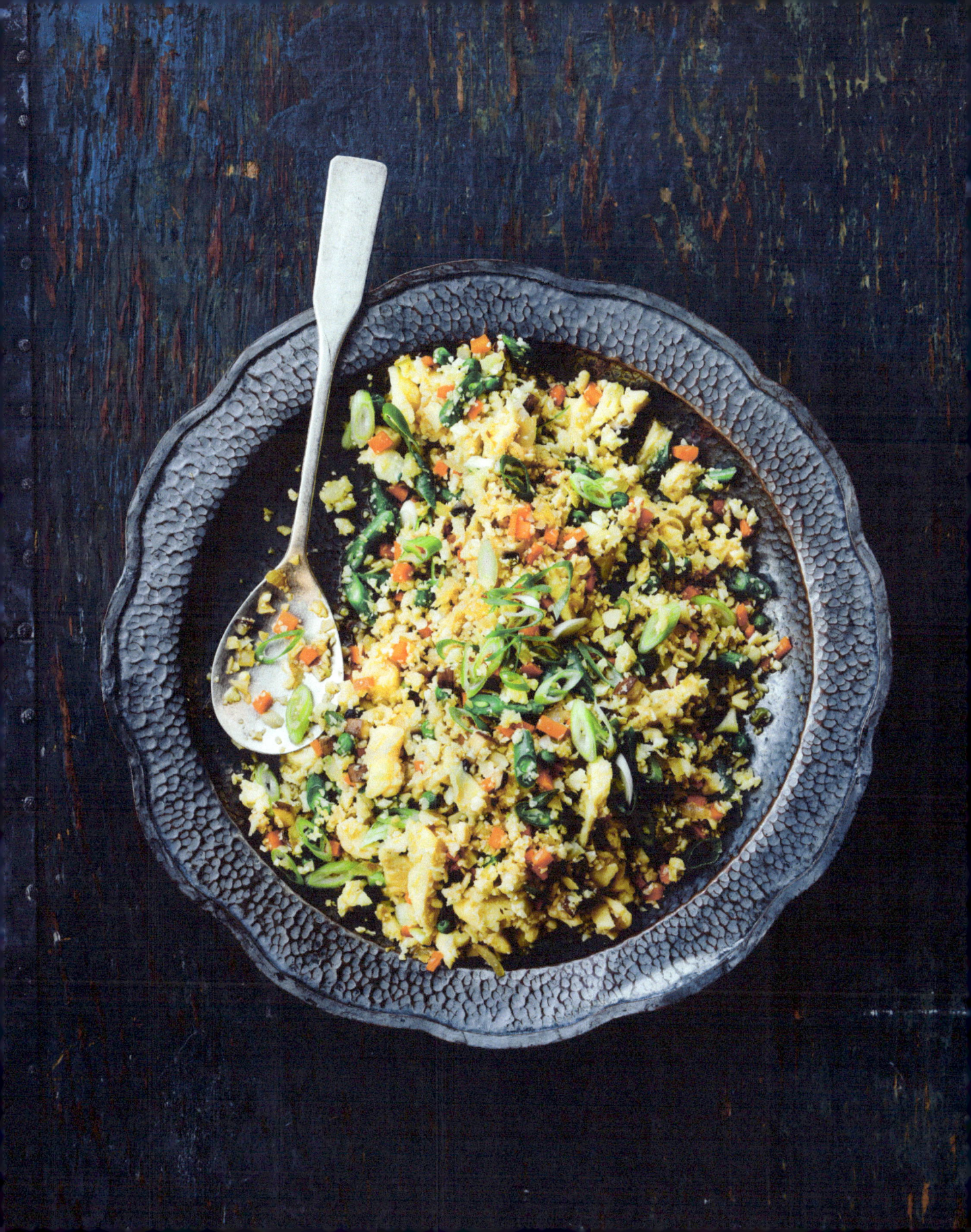

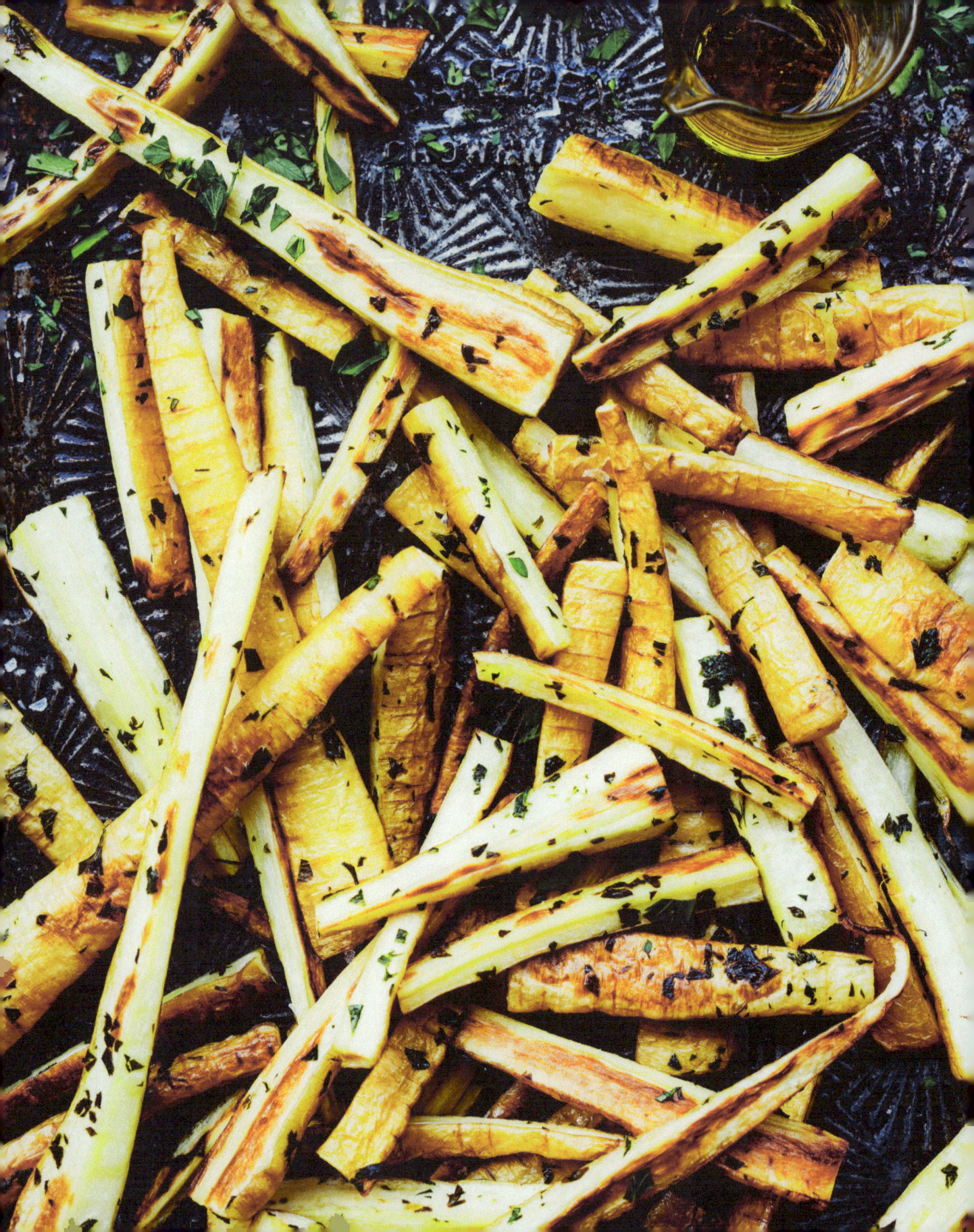

PARSNIP FRIES

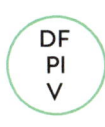

DF
PI
V

A fun way to get to know parsnips is to make them into French fries. They are more nutritionally dense than potatoes, but still hold a similar consistency. On their own, parsnips have a nice warming spiced flavor but also take on additional flavors well. Cooking them to where they are brown on the outside but soft on the inside makes for a very satisfying Paleo alternative to potato fries.

Serves 4 to 6

3 tablespoons extra-virgin olive oil

2 tablespoons chopped fresh parsley

8 medium parsnips, peeled and cut into fries

Sea salt to taste

Truffle oil, for drizzling (optional)

1. Preheat the oven to 400°F.

2. Whisk together the olive oil and parsley in a mixing bowl. Add the parsnip fries, toss to coat, and season with salt.

3. Spread the fries out on a large baking sheet. Bake for 15 minutes, or until the fries are lightly browned on one side.

4. Remove from the oven flip the fries over with a large spatula. Increase the oven temperature to 450°F. Bake for an additional 5 minutes until crispy and lightly browned on both sides.

5. Serve hot drizzled with truffle oil, if using, or with your favorite dipping sauce (see Tip).

TIP

These fries are great dipped in our Dairy-Free Ranch Dressing (page 74), Arugula Sunflower Pesto (page 40), or even our Whole-Egg Mayonnaise (page 90).

CHOPPED ROASTED VEGGIES

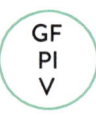

GF
PI
V

These veggies are packed with flavor and make a great accompaniment to any main dish or your salad greens. We also like to use them as part of an antipasti plate with meats and cheeses.

Makes about 4 cups

2½ tablespoons extra-virgin olive oil

1½ teaspoons maple syrup

1½ teaspoons balsamic vinegar

¼ teaspoon dried oregano

4 cups assorted chopped vegetables in 1-inch pieces (asparagus, onion, parsnips, mushrooms, rutabagas, green zucchini, yellow squash, halved grape tomatoes are all great options)

Sea salt to taste

1. Preheat the oven to 375°F.

2. Whisk together the oil, maple syrup, and vinegar and oregano in a small bowl.

3. Put the chopped veggies in a large bowl. Pour the dressing over the vegetables and stir to coat.

4. Spread out the veggies in a roasting pan and bake uncovered for 30 minutes, stirring once during the cooking time. Season with salt.

5. Serve hot or at room temperature.

TIP

This recipe is versatile. You can use almost any vegetables you have on hand, or whatever you find in season at your local market.

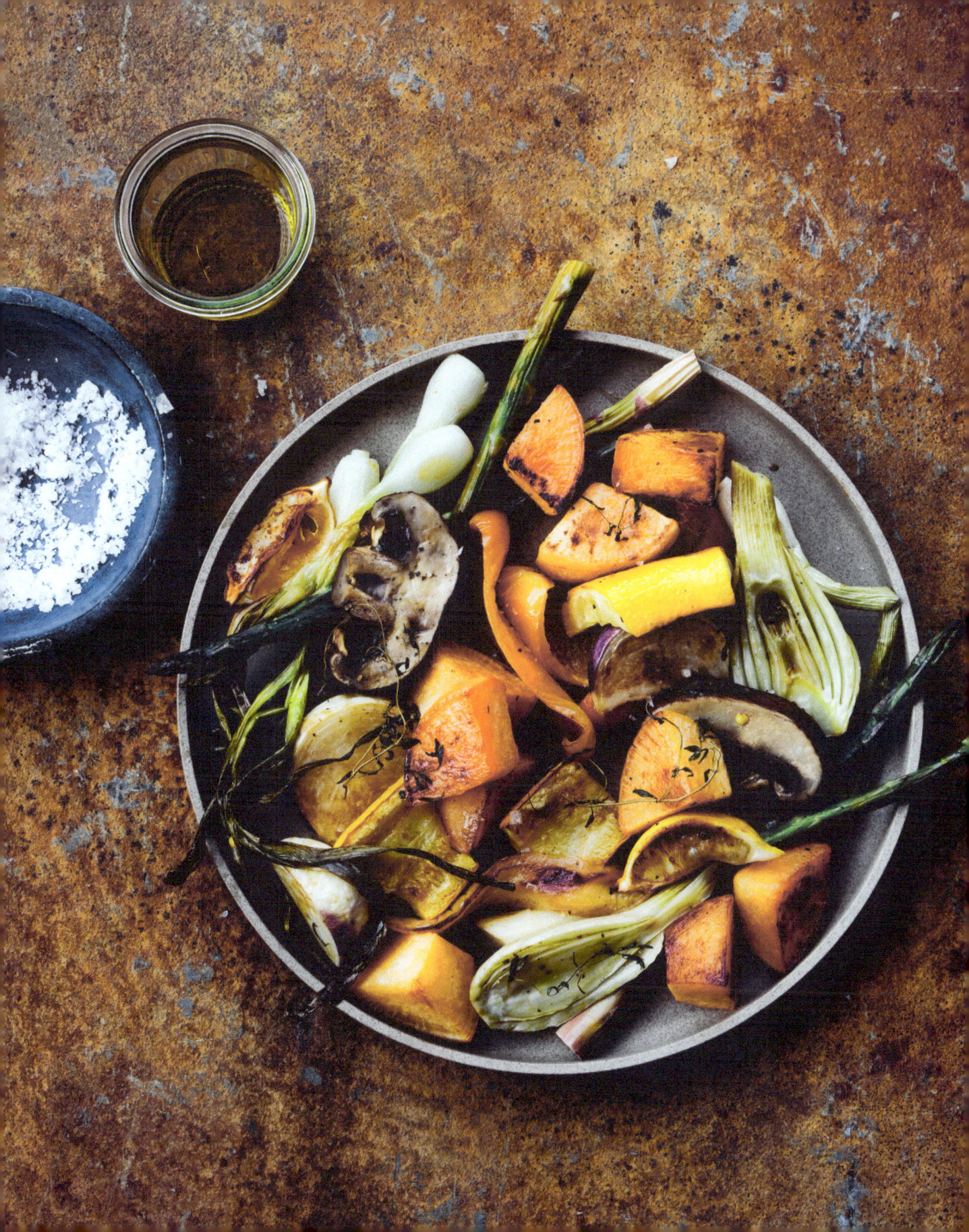

"CREAMED" KALE

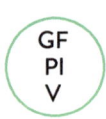

GF
PI
V

This is our dairy-free take on creamed spinach. We took out the cream and added cashews, miso, and nutritional yeast to make it a super-nutritious and delicious side dish. We enjoy this served with any grilled or seared seafood or on its own for a hearty protein-rich vegan dish.

Serves 4 to 6

2 large bunches of kale, de-stemmed and chopped into bite sized pieces (see Tip)

2 tablespoons fresh lemon juice

Sea salt to taste

½ cup vegetable broth

¼ onion, finely chopped

1 clove garlic, minced

1½ cups full-fat canned coconut milk

¾ cup raw cashews, covered in water and simmered for 30 minutes, then drained

¼ cup nutritional yeast

2 tablespoons white miso

Pinch of freshly grated nutmeg

½ tablespoon coconut oil

1. Put the chopped kale in a mixing bowl with the lemon juice and a pinch of salt. Rub the kale between your hands for a few minutes, massaging the leaves until they have a silky texture. Set aside.

2. Heat the broth in a small pot over medium heat. Add the onion and garlic and cook until softened, 5 to 7 minutes.

3. Transfer the seasoned broth to a blender or food processor. Add the coconut milk, cashews, nutritional yeast, miso, and nutmeg and puree until smooth.

4. In a medium sauté pan, heat the coconut oil and sauté the kale until fully cooked. Add the coconut milk mixture and reduce until the sauce has thickened.

5. Serve immediately. The final product should be loose but not soupy.

TIP

Spinach or Swiss chard can be substituted for kale in this recipe.

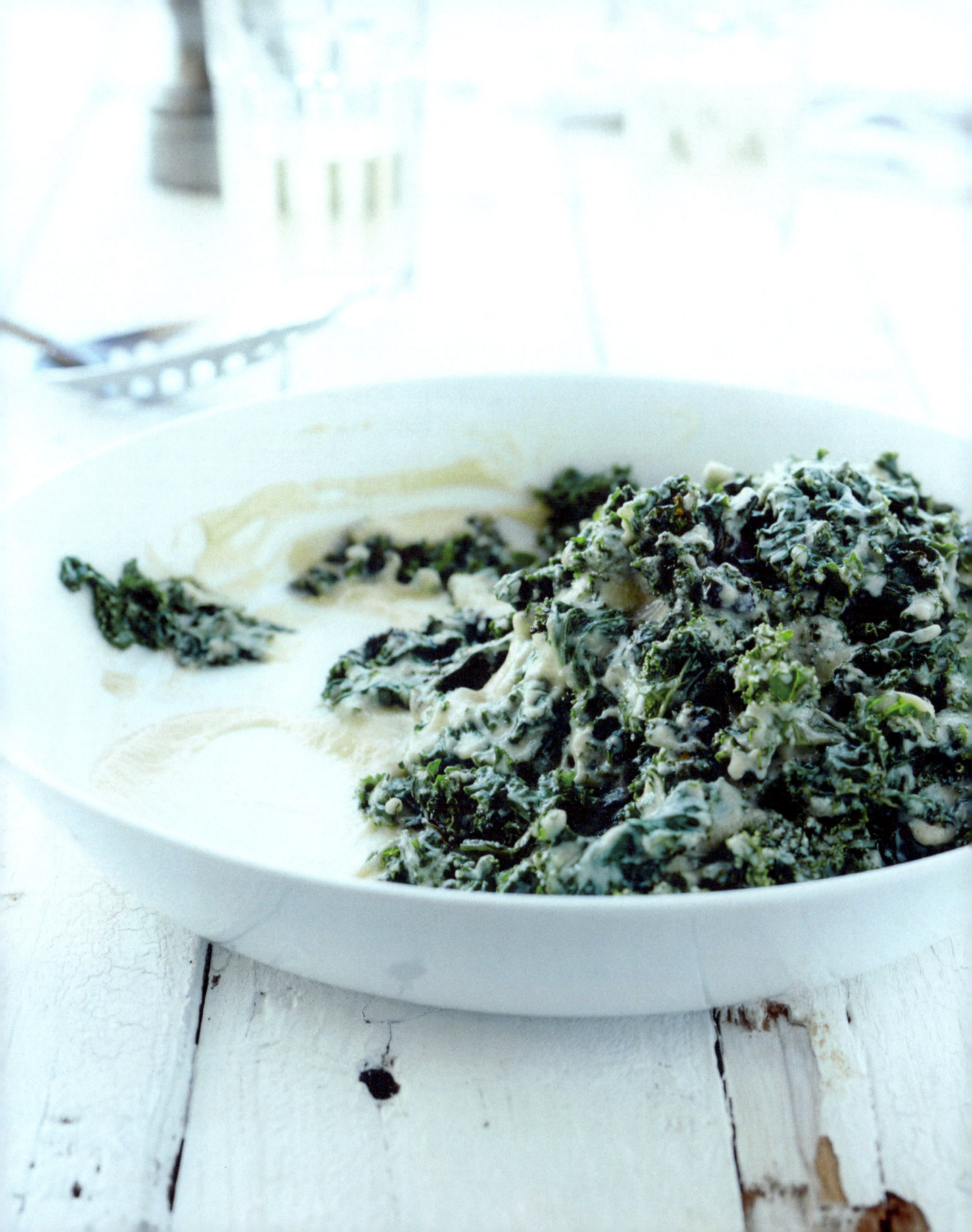

DAIRY-FREE MAC & CHEESE

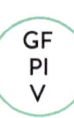

If using
spaghetti
squash

**GF
PI
V**

This dairy-free version of mac and cheese is creamy and luscious. We love using nutritional yeast, which is highly nutritious and easily found in powder or flakes at a natural grocer. The yeast acts as the "cheezy" component here, (and we also enjoy sprinkling it on popcorn or eggs!).

Serves 4 to 6

1 pound brown rice
pasta or quinoa pasta
(we like shells or elbows)
or Baked Spaghetti
Squash (page 118)

2 cups full-fat canned
coconut milk

1½ cups nutritional yeast,
plus more for sprinkling

Pinch of paprika, for color

¼ teaspoon sea salt,
plus more to taste

1. Cook the pasta as directed on the package.

2. Meanwhile, in a saucepan on medium heat, bring the canned coconut milk, nutritional yeast, paprika, and salt to a rolling boil, then reduce the heat to low and simmer for 5 minutes, until all of the ingredients are incorporated and the sauce is creamy and smooth. Remove from the heat and set aside.

3. When the pasta is ready, drain and rinse it well. Add the pasta to the sauce, tossing to coat. Season with more salt, if needed, and simmer the mac and cheese on low heat for another 2 minutes.

4. Sprinkle with additional nutritional yeast and serve immediately.

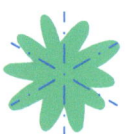

TIP

To make this a heartier main dish, we often add 12 ounces of cooked grass-fed ground beef or turkey for added protein.

Jennifer: When I want a comforting dish this is my go to. I do not eat much dairy. For me, too much of it makes my nose stuffed up and slows my digestion. But when I have dairy only occasionally, my body digests it more easily. This dish fully satiates my cravings for creamy dairy every time.

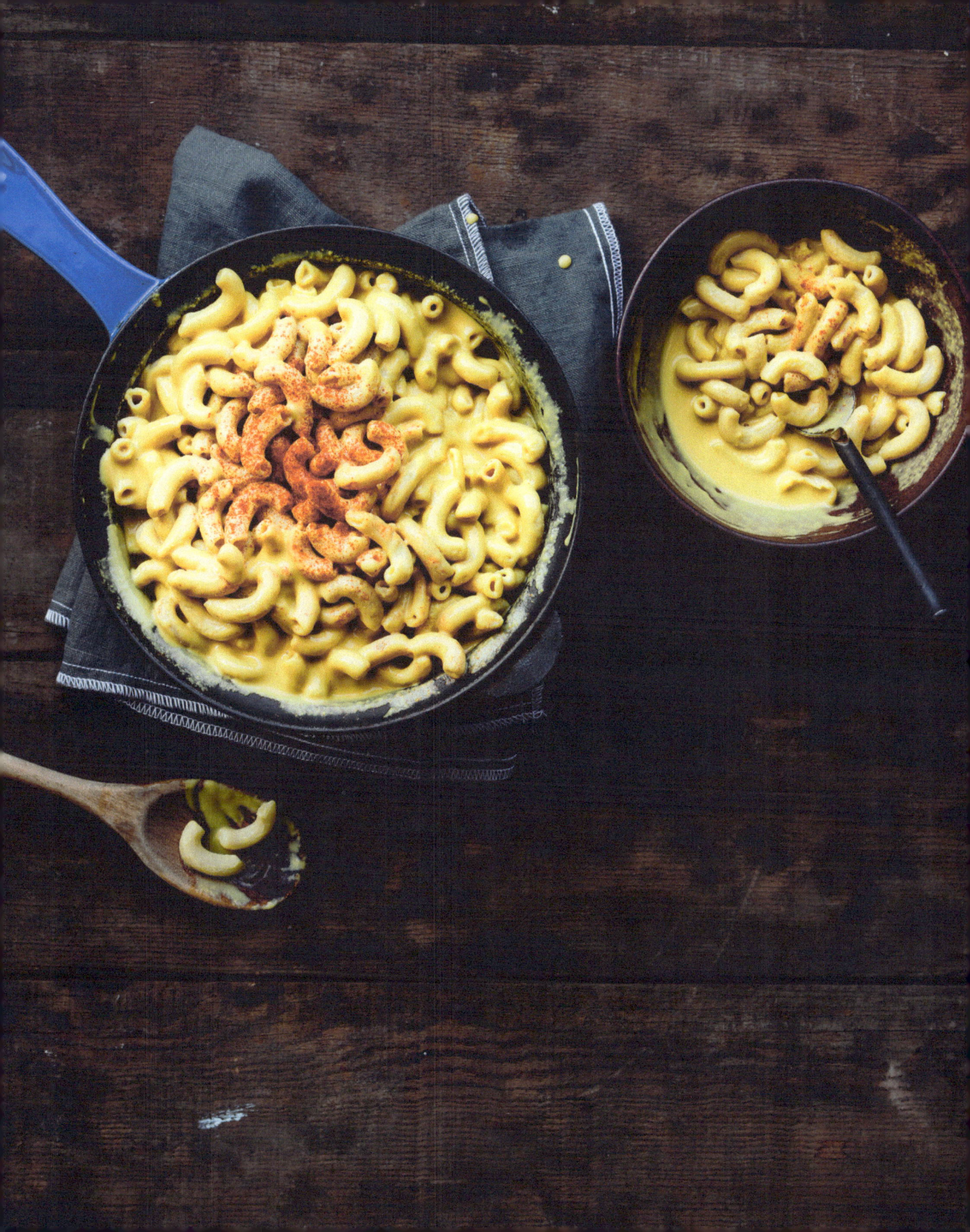

BAKED MAC & CHEESE WITH CAULIFLOWER

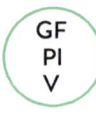

If using spaghetti squash

GF
PI
V

Because cauliflower is mild in flavor, this is a perfect way to sneak in some veggies and added fiber for you and your kids: Baking cauliflower with cheese and pasta is the perfect disguise. This recipe has been a family favorite for years. Here is our gluten-free version.

Serves 4 to 6

10 ounces brown rice elbow or penne pasta, or Baked Spaghetti Squash (page 118)

4 tablespoons unsalted butter

3 tablespoons brown rice flour

2 tablespoons mustard powder

3 cups milk

3 cups shredded cheddar cheese

3 cups cauliflower, chopped into small pieces and steamed for 5 minutes

Sea salt to taste

½ cup Pecorino Romano cheese, grated

½ cup gluten-free breadcrumbs (page 91)

¼ cup crispy crumbled bacon (optional)

1. Preheat the oven to 350°F.

2. Cook the pasta as directed on the package. Drain and rinse it well. Toss in 2 tablespoons of the butter and set the pasta aside.

3. Melt the remaining 2 tablespoons butter in a large pot on medium-low heat. Gradually add the flour and mustard, whisking constantly for about two minutes to make a roux.

4. Gradually add the milk, still whisking constantly, until a sauce forms, approximately 4 minutes. Add the cheddar and whisk until it melts into the sauce.

5. Add the steamed cauliflower and stir to coat. Add the pasta and stir to cover with the cheese sauce and cauliflower. Season with salt.

6. Pour into a baking dish and top with the Pecorino, breadcrumbs, and bacon if using. Bake for approximately 10 minutes, until it is hot and the top is golden brown and crispy.

7. Let rest for 5 minutes before serving.

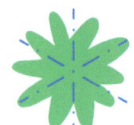

TIP

You can play around with different cheeses, such as goat cheese or Gruyère. You can also use other vegetables: We have made this with cooked winter or summer squash (or broccoli) in place of the cauliflower.

GLUTEN-FREE PIZZA CRUST

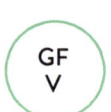

GF
V

There are a lot of gluten-free pizza dough recipes out there, but we believe our take on it is one of the easiest, tastiest, and home-cook friendliest. Because of our Italian roots, pizza has always equaled celebration! We throw pizza parties with friends featuring this crust and lots of wine, and kid parties where each little one gets to create, eat, and share their own pizza pie.

Makes two 12-inch pizza crusts

1 cup warm water (105°F to 110°F)

1 packet (¼ ounce) active dry yeast (about 1½ teaspoons)

2 tablespoons honey

2 tablespoons flax seeds

¼ cup room temperature water

1 cup tapioca starch

¾ cup potato starch

1¾ cups brown rice flour, plus more for dusting

½ cup millet flour

3 teaspoons baking powder

2 teaspoons xanthan gum

1 teaspoon fine sea salt, plus more for seasoning

¼ cup extra-virgin olive oil, plus extra for the pan and the top of pizza

¼ teaspoon apple cider vinegar

1. Grease two 12-inch pizza pans and dust lightly with brown rice flour. Set aside.

2. In a small bowl, combine the warm water and yeast, mixing thoroughly. Addthe honey and mix thoroughly. Let sit for 5 to 10 minutes, until the yeast mixture starts to foam.

3. Meanwhile, combine the flax and room temperature water together and set aside for 5 minutes.

4. In a large mixing bowl, whisk together the tapioca and potato starches, the brown rice and millet flours, the baking powder, xanthan gum, and salt. Add the reserved flax mixture, olive oil, and cider vinegar and mix. The pizza dough should be creamy and smooth with a consistency similar to cake batter.

5. Using a rubber spatula, divide the dough in half. Scoop each half onto the center of a greased pizza pan. Using wet hands, press down lightly and flatten the dough to create a thin, even, round pizza shell with slightly raised edges. (Keep wetting your hands to make this easier, and take your time to smooth out the dough.)

6. Preheat the oven to 400°F. Put the pizza shells in a warm spot to rest and rise a bit, about 15 minutes.

7. When the oven is hot, bake the two pizzas, side by side on the center rack, for 15 minutes or until golden. (If your oven is too small to accommodate both pans on one rack, use two racks, rotating the pans halfway through baking time to avoid overcooking on the lower rack).

8. Remove the baked pizza shells from the oven. Preheat the broiler.

9. Brush the warm pizza shells with olive oil and season with salt. Top with your choice of sauce, cheese, cooked vegetables, fresh herbs, and/or meat. Drizzle olive oil all over the tops. Broil the pizzas briefly to melt the cheese, 4 to 5 minutes. They are best served right out of the broiler.

TIP

If you only want one pizza, you can either halve the dough recipe or refrigerate half of the prepared dough for up to 2 days. Yeasted doughs do not freeze well because a deep freeze may kill the yeast. Even if we want just one pizza, we usually just make two and enjoy the leftovers, hot or cold.

GRAIN-FREE PIZZA CRUST

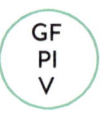

GF
PI
V

This pizza dough may surprise you! It has an unusual list of ingredients and yet it bakes off beautifully. The crispy crust satisfies the Paleo person who is craving a pizza. It can also be used as a flatbread.

Makes one 12-inch pizza crust

About half a head of cauliflower, outer leaves removed

1 large egg

Pinch of sea salt,

1 tablespoon dried oregano (optional)

1 cup plus 3 tablespoons tapioca starch/flour

¼ cup extra-virgin olive oil, plus more for drizzling

1 tablespoon warm water

1. Preheat the oven to 400*F.

2. In a food processor or by hand with a grater, shred the cauliflower until you have ⅓ cup.

3. In a small covered saucepan over medium-low heat, steam the cauliflower in about ¼ cup water until soft, approximately 6 minutes. Drain in a small, fine mesh or nut strainer bag, squeezing out as much excess water as possible.

4. Whisk the egg in a mixing bowl. Add the cooked and drained cauliflower, the pinch of salt, and oregano, if using, and mix to combine. Add the tapioca flour, mixing until thoroughly incorporated. Add the olive oil and warm water. Mix by hand to create a dough, then shape into a ball. The dough can be wrapped and frozen at this point or put in the refrigerator to be used with in 2 days.

5. Place the ball of dough between two pieces of 9 x 11-inch parchment paper. Flatten the ball with your hand. Using a rolling pin, roll out the dough to create a 12-inch round. Slowly peel off the top piece of parchment paper. Carefully flip the remaining piece of parchment over so that your dough is on your pizza stone, pizza pan, or a cookie sheet.

6. Top with your choice of sauce, cheese, cooked vegetables, fresh herbs, and/ or meat and bake for 15-18 minutes or until crust is golden brown. This pizza is best served right out of the oven with a drizzle of olive oil on top.

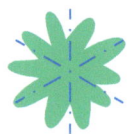

TIP

If you do not have parchment paper, wet the rolling pin with water to keep the dough from sticking to the pin. (It should be damp but not dripping.) You'll find the dough easier to roll out.

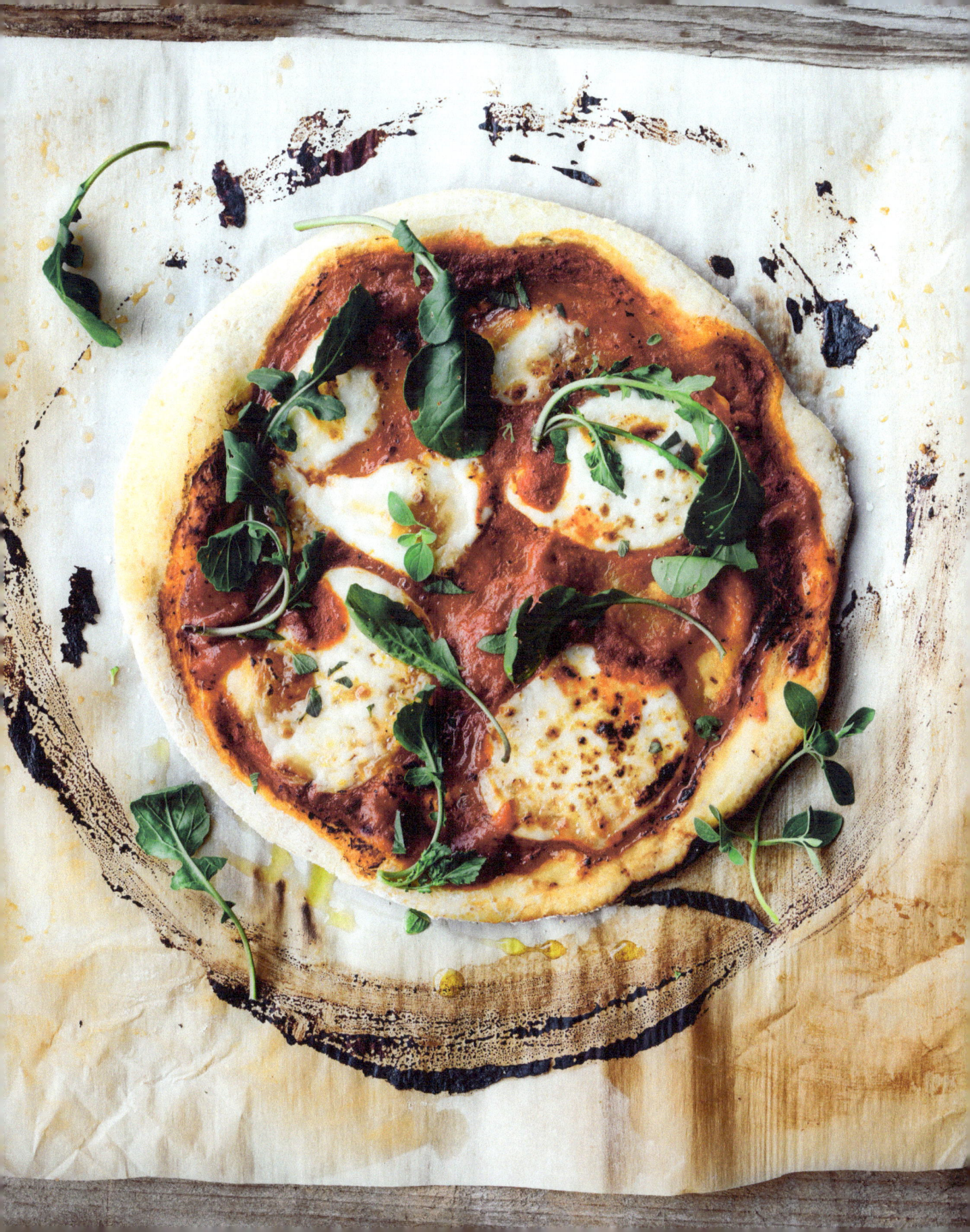

GET YOUR BOOGIE ON

MOVEMENT MEDICINE

Jill: Movement medicine is truly one of the highs of my life. I love feeling my body because I learn so much about myself through it. I love finding new rhythms within, discovering new music and creating choreography to share with people that helps free our mind, body, and soul. Our body holds our deepest wisdom and, when the energy flows freely, we heal stuck places emotionally and physically, we strengthen our intuition and our inner power, and we gain a stronger sense of who we are and what we came here to do.

It is so simple and so profound. This is why we created Shine Living Community, where we lead unique varieties of movement medicine for all ages and levels of dance, yoga, meditation, breathwork, warrior workouts, and our Freedom Movement Method. Movement is primal and when we move and raise our energy together, we not only heal ourselves, but we heal our family systems, our communities, humanity, and our planet. You are that powerful!

So, let's get moving. Oh, and if you think you can't dance? I beg to differ—we all have our own

unique rhythm. All it takes is curiosity, courage and willingness. So, let's get moving! Join our live and live stream classes from anywhere on the planet at shinelivingcommunity.com.

Choose activities you enjoy: If you love to run, great, DO IT! If you feel dread every time you lace up your running shoes, by all means find something else. There are a million things you can do to get

your heart rate up, so by golly do something you enjoy! If you aren't sure what that is, take some classes and experiment. Think outside the box.

Change it up: It is good for your body to use different muscles, so mixing it up is not only beneficial and gets maximum results but will keep you from getting bored. Yoga one day, running, the next, biking, dance, hiking with a friend, whatever gets you excited on that particular day is what you should do. Listen to what your body wants and go with that.

Get outside: There is nothing like getting out in nature to get connected to our bodies. Not only does the outdoors tend to provide us with a more strenuous platform because of the variety of surfaces, but it also keeps things interesting. Rather than biking or running on something stationary and staring at the same thing the whole time, fresh air can revitalize us and reduce stress. Many of us stare at screens all day long, so it is beneficial to let nature be your exercise companion.

Pair up with a friend or a group: A wonderful option is to join our global Shine Living Community to share in a wide variety of classes the whole family will LOVE. Having a hard time getting motivated? Exercise with friends! It is a great way to catch up. When you exercise with friends or a group, you hold each other accountable and you can be each other's cheerleader. For some people, signing up for group exercise activities is what gets them to stick to it. If that sounds like you, then look into local meet-up groups for activities or sign up for some classes. If you are a goaloriented person, maybe a group race that has a training schedule leading up to the event will work for you. If that is what it takes, get going!

Commit: Even if you do just 30 minutes most days, you will feel the difference. Make getting a little exercise part of your daily routine and stick to it. Think of it as a gift to yourself, to your health, and to your vitality—and something that feeds every single aspect of your life. You deserve to feel amazing and exercise will absolutely help achieve that.

Take time to wind down, stretch, and give gratitude: Exercise increases dopamine, serotonin, and endorphins in your body—all-natural, feel-good enhancers. Just as beneficial as the workout is taking in some long deep breaths as you stretch and give gratitude for that beautiful body of yours that is strong and able.

It is in our nature to move. We weren't built to sit in front of computers all day. Our bodies need to release through movement, to stretch, and to work our muscles to remain healthy. Exercise affects brain health and the immune system, it oxygenates our cells, and delivers a ton of other benefits. Boogie on with your fabulous self!

Jill: Moving my body is truly one of the highs of my life. I absolutely LOVE to dance and love leading others in dance where we experience transforming energy and building strength, stamina and joy together through somatic choreography, music and inspired community. Dance keeps our bodies and brain young and vibrant. it opens us to new parts of ourselves and to a higher perspective on our life path because when we raise our energy we start to see solutions where we once felt stuck. It is incredible medicine and it is a real good time too!

Jessica: My yoga and meditation practice has been an anchor point in my life. It helps to awaken to my own inner compass instead of looking outside of me for the answers or for what it should look like. It has also helped me heal my body and awaken my spirit on so many levels. I love leading and practicing yoga and meditation in community because when we practice together, the energy amplifies (it has been measured!) and we not only heal ourselves, but our families, our communities, and the planet. I consider practicing on the mat (and on the dance floor) together an incredible act of service. It can and will change your life and the life of those around you. So let's practice....

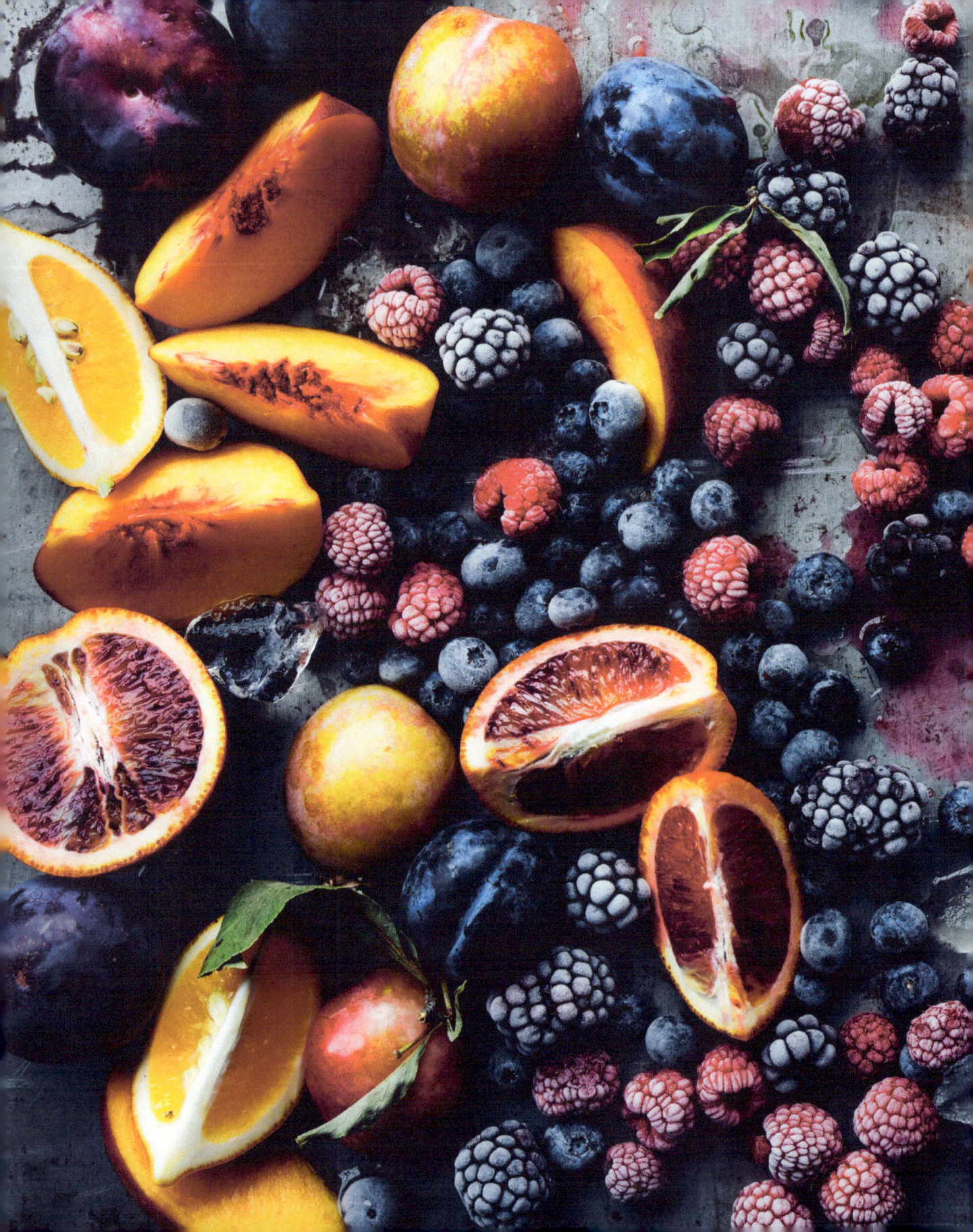

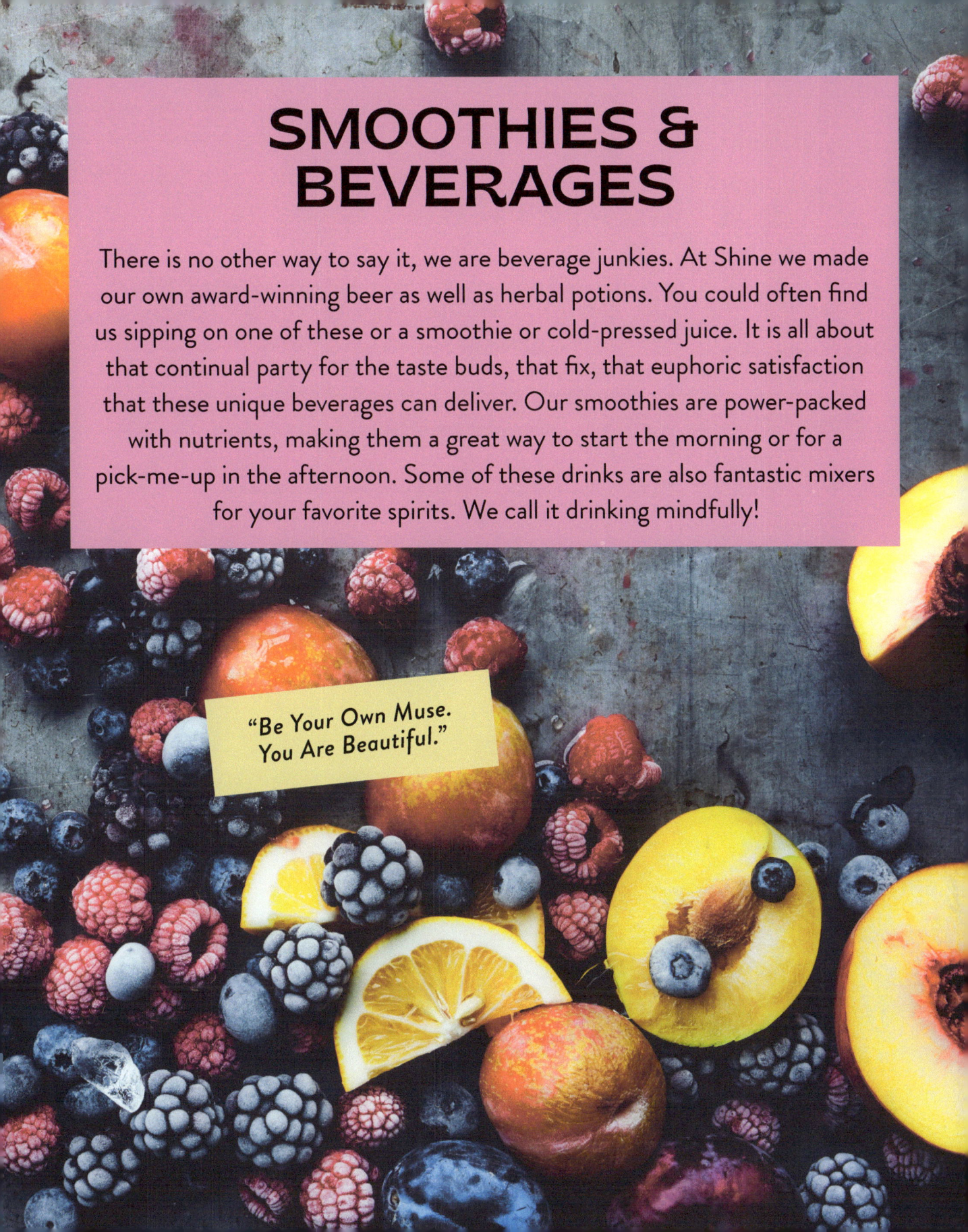

SMOOTHIES & BEVERAGES

There is no other way to say it, we are beverage junkies. At Shine we made our own award-winning beer as well as herbal potions. You could often find us sipping on one of these or a smoothie or cold-pressed juice. It is all about that continual party for the taste buds, that fix, that euphoric satisfaction that these unique beverages can deliver. Our smoothies are power-packed with nutrients, making them a great way to start the morning or for a pick-me-up in the afternoon. Some of these drinks are also fantastic mixers for your favorite spirits. We call it drinking mindfully!

"Be Your Own Muse.
You Are Beautiful."

NETTLE & MINT ICED TEA

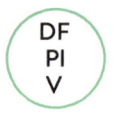

**DF
PI
V**

***Makes three
8-ounce servings***

3 cups filtered water

3 tablespoons dried
nettles (see Tip)

1 tablespoon dried
peppermint

1 lemon

1 to 2 tablespoons
raw honey

1. Bring the filtered water to a boil. Put the nettles and peppermint into a quart-sized mason jar. Pour the boiling water over the herbs and stir in the honey. Cover and let sit overnight at room temperature.

2. The next day, strain your tea into a pitcher full of ice. Let it sit for 30 minutes to allow some of the ice to melt.

3. Cut the lemon in half. Juice one half and pour the juice into the pitcher. Slice the other half.

4. Serve the tea over ice. Garnish each glass with a lemon slice.

TIP

Properly dried nettles will usually maintain their stinging sensation. If this is a concern, use kitchen gloves to handle the nettles. If you like, add lavender or dandelion leaf during the last 2 to 3 hours of steeping to increase the health benefits and vary the flavor.

Jessica: *I made this tea often while I was pregnant and roasting hot in the height of summer. Not only is it extremely nourishing for both mama and baby, it is cooling and rejuvenating. Even if you are not pregnant, summer heat can be fun but also irritating at times. Drink up!*

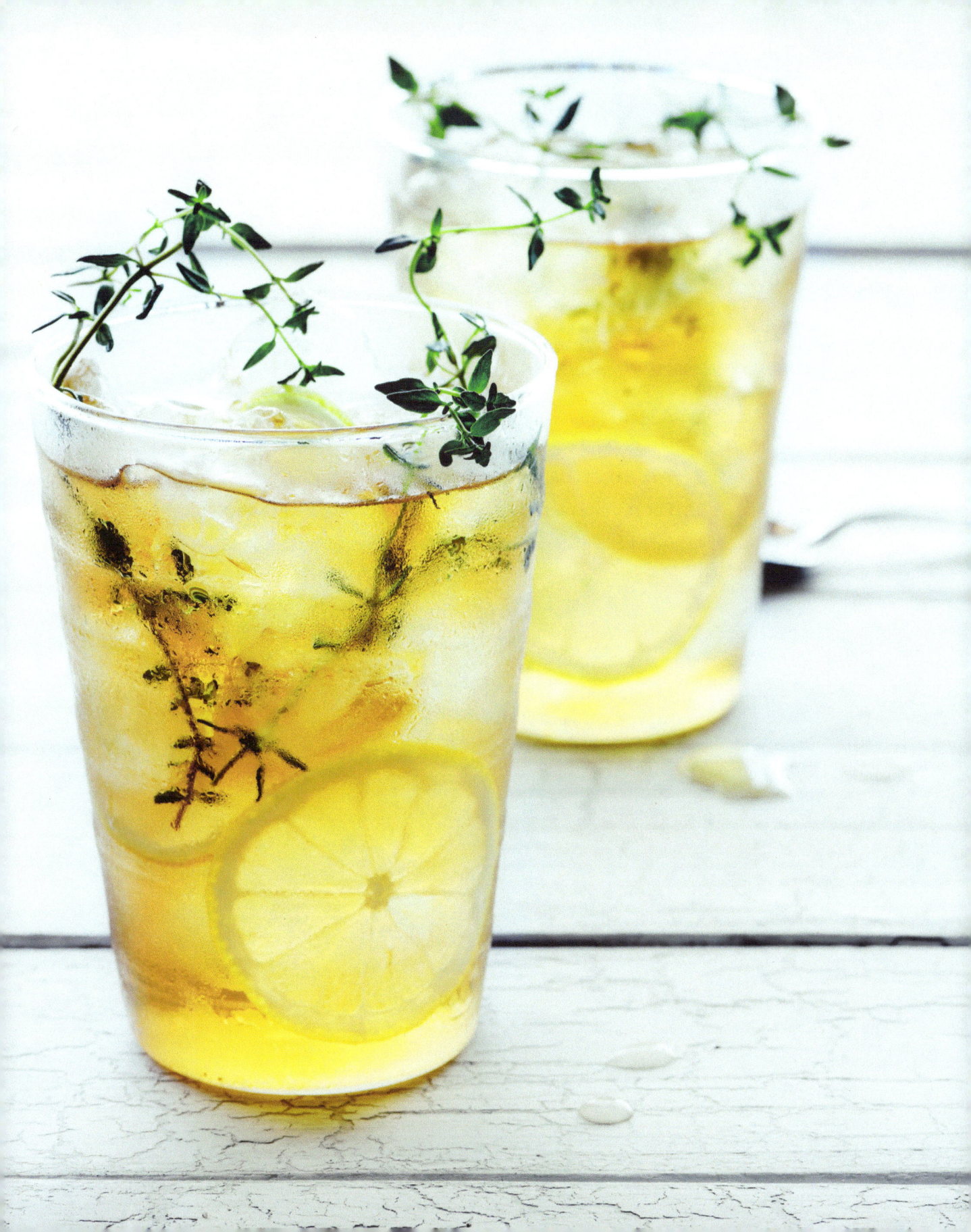

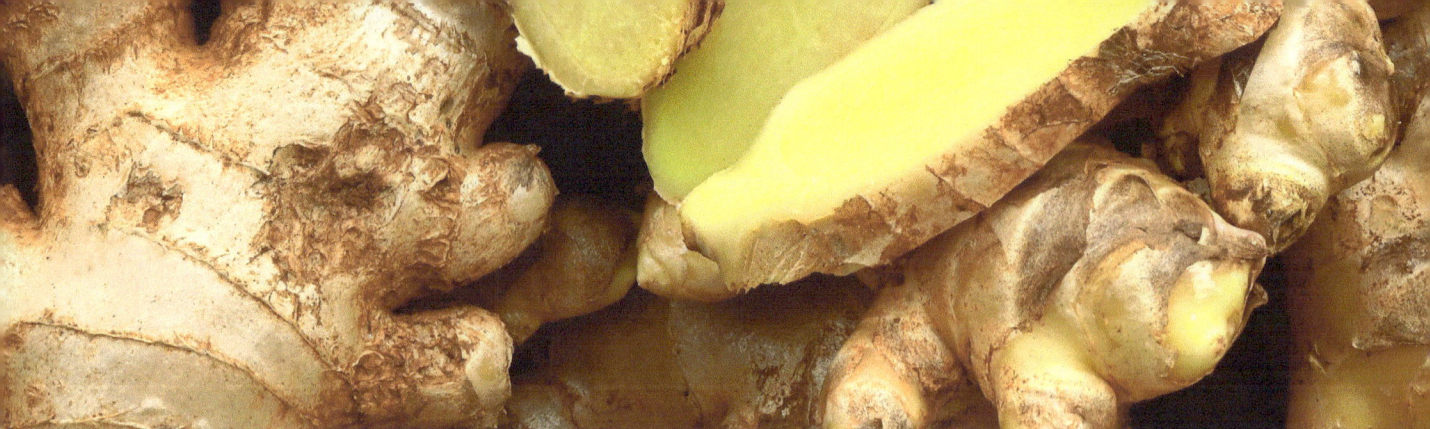

FRESH GINGER ALE

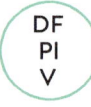
DF
PI
V

Makes 1 quart
¼ cup fresh lemon juice
1 quart filtered water,
at room temperature
¼ cup filtered water
2 heaping tablespoons
grated ginger
1 tablespoon raw honey
2 cups sparkling water.

1. Add the lemon juice, water, honey and fresh ginger to a high powered blender and blend for about 30 seconds.

2. Strain the blended liquid through a fine strainer.

3. Put the strained liquid into 2 glasses (2 ounces in each).

4. Add 1 cup of carbonated liquid to each cup and stir. Add ice or serve as is.

Jessica: This drink is refreshing and health boosting. Ginger is wonderful for circulation and digestion. The raw honey is high in antioxidants as well as a great boost for brain power. I love drinking this mid-day during our retreats and workshops or before I pick up the kids from school. It's like an "Oh, yes I can!" in a glass.

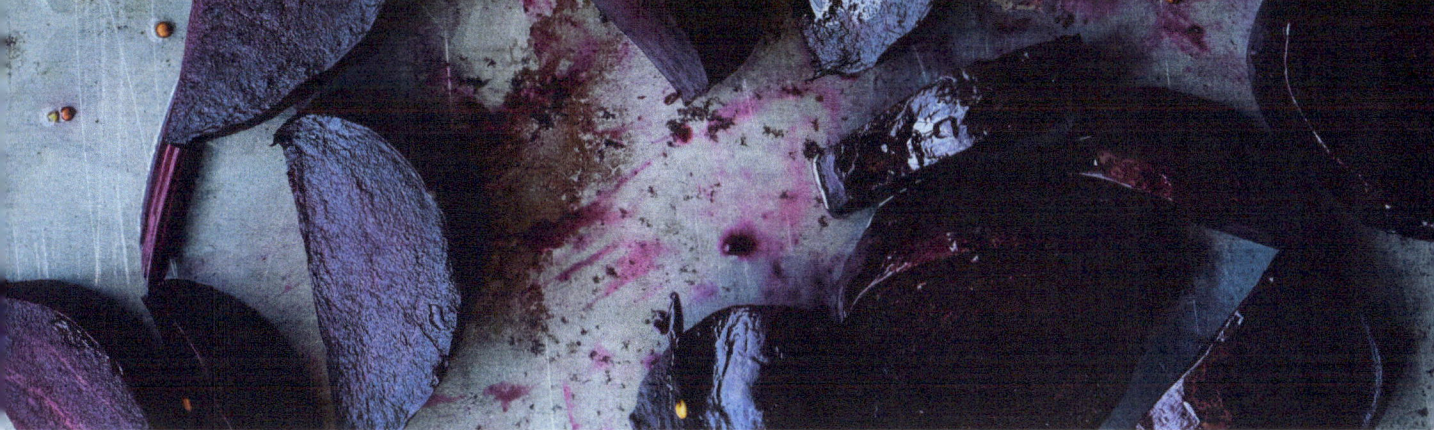

BEET KVASS

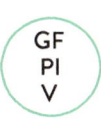

GF
PI
V

Kvass is a traditional Eastern European medicinal tonic with an earthy, salty taste that's very cleansing for the liver and beneficial for healthy digestion. You can drink it or use it in place of vinegar in salad dressings. We really enjoy sipping this before or after meals, served chilled in a wineglass.

Makes two 10-ounce servings

3 medium beets, peels on

1 tablespoon sea salt

about ½ gallon filtered water

1. Wash the beets to remove the dirt. (Be careful not to scrub too hard; you want the beneficial bacteria to remain, as it is a crucial part of the fermentation process.)

2. Chop the beets into medium pieces and place them in a clean half-gallon mason jar. Add the sea salt and fill the jar with filtered water, making sure to leave ½-inch of headspace. Tightly screw on the lid, turn the jar upside down, and give a light shake to incorporate the ingredients.

3. Let the beverage ferment at room temperature, on your countertop, for approximately 2 weeks (see Tip). Taste it: If it has a deep, earthy, pickle-like flavor, it's ready. It could take a few days longer, depending on the temperature of your kitchen.

4. When the flavor of the kvass is where you would like it, store it in the refrigerator for up to 1 month. It is great as a digestif or really any time of day. There is no need to strain out the beets. You can even eat them as they get poured out into your glass.

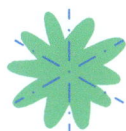

TIP

Make sure to "burp" your jar every day for the first 3 or 4 days of the fermentation process to let the gas escape. Do this by removing the cap for a couple of seconds and then securely twisting it back on. If it's available, the best way to make beet kvass is with raw grass-fed whey (rather than the water and salt). Whey is the watery part of raw milk that remains after the formation of curds. It reduces the fermentation time and adds a sour flavor to kvass.

WATERMELON COOLER

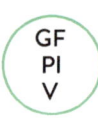

GF
PI
V

Watermelon seeds are very nourishing for the kidneys, which can get taxed during long, high-energy summer days, and are even rich in minerals and great for healthy hair and skin. We recommend blending them right in with the rest of the watermelon. Watermelons with seeds tend to be more flavorful.

Makes about two 10-ounce servings

2 cups bite-sized pieces of ripe watermelon

3 cups full-fat canned coconut milk

1 cup ice cubes

sea salt to taste

Place all of the ingredients in a blender and blend for approximately 2 minutes, until cool and creamy. Serve immediately.

TIP

If you don't have coconut milk in the house, you can substitute filtered water or coconut water for a frothy watermelon beverage, served straight up.

Jennifer: I love watermelon and I love coconut milk, so having them together as a beverage is deeply satisfying. I often drink this at the end of the day, in the late-summer sun, while swinging in my hammock. Watermelon is mostly made of water, so it is very cooling and hydrating to the body.

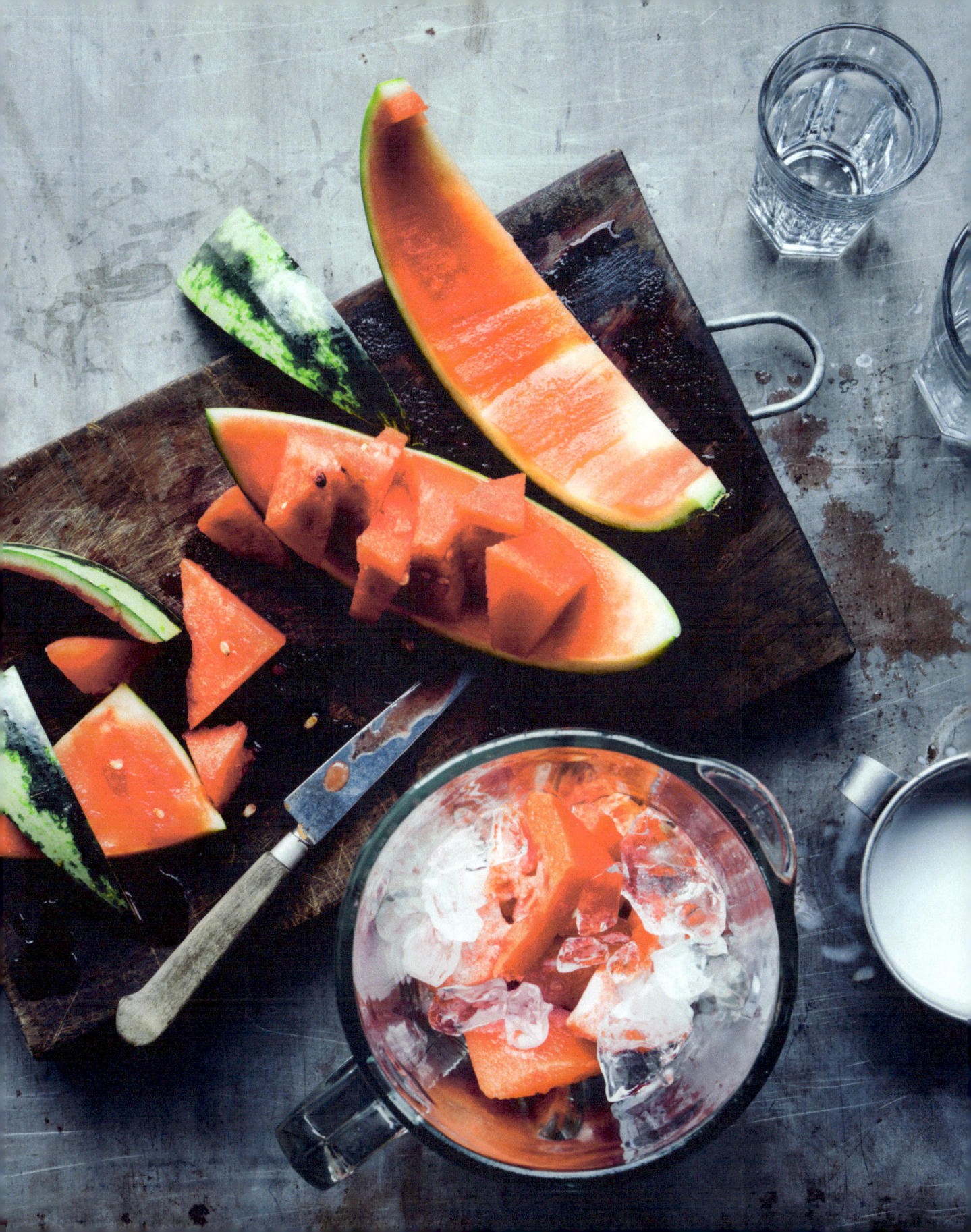

SUMMER LOVIN' ELIXIR

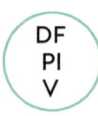

Chill out in the heat of summer with the cooling power of cucumbers, lime, and mint. Blended together with a burst of healthy leafy greens and more, this drink is the ultimate refresher.

Makes about two 10-ounce servings

1 small cucumber, peeled

Flesh of ½ avocado

2 teaspoons fresh lime juice

2 teaspoons fresh mint

1 cup chopped greens of your choice (spinach, beet greens, Swiss chard, or kale), lightly steamed (see Tip)

1 cup distilled water (see Tip)

2 cups ice cubes

Put all of the ingredients in a blender and blend for approximately 2 minutes, until smooth. Serve immediately.

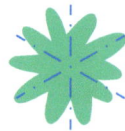

TIP

Lightly steaming the greens makes them easier to digest and all of the nutrients more readily available. Coconut water can be exchanged for the water for added electrolytes and sweetness.

GOLDEN ANTI-INFLAMMATORY SMOOTHIE

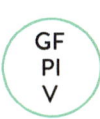

GF
PI
V

Turmeric is revered around the world as one of the world's most powerful antiinflammatory foods. However, its highly beneficial compounds can be hard to absorb without the presence of fat or black pepper. We know it sounds strange to include black pepper in a smoothie, but the flavor is masked and the benefits of doing so are worth it. This drink is truly so good for you and tastes amazing as well.

Makes about two 10-ounce servings

2 teaspoons chia seeds

2 cups full-fat canned coconut milk

2 tablespoons powdered turmeric

¼ teaspoon ground black pepper

2 teaspoons raw cacao

½ teaspoon fresh ginger, minced

2 cups frozen mango or frozen banana

2 tablespoons coconut oil

2 tablespoons raw honey

2 cups ice cubes

Soak the chia seeds in the coconut milk in the blender for approximately 10 minutes (see Tip). Add the remaining ingredients to the blender and blend for approximately 1 minute, until smooth. Serve immediately. Serve immediately. The final product should be loose but not soupy.

TIP

Soaking the chia seeds in liquid before blending enhances the digestibility of the seeds.

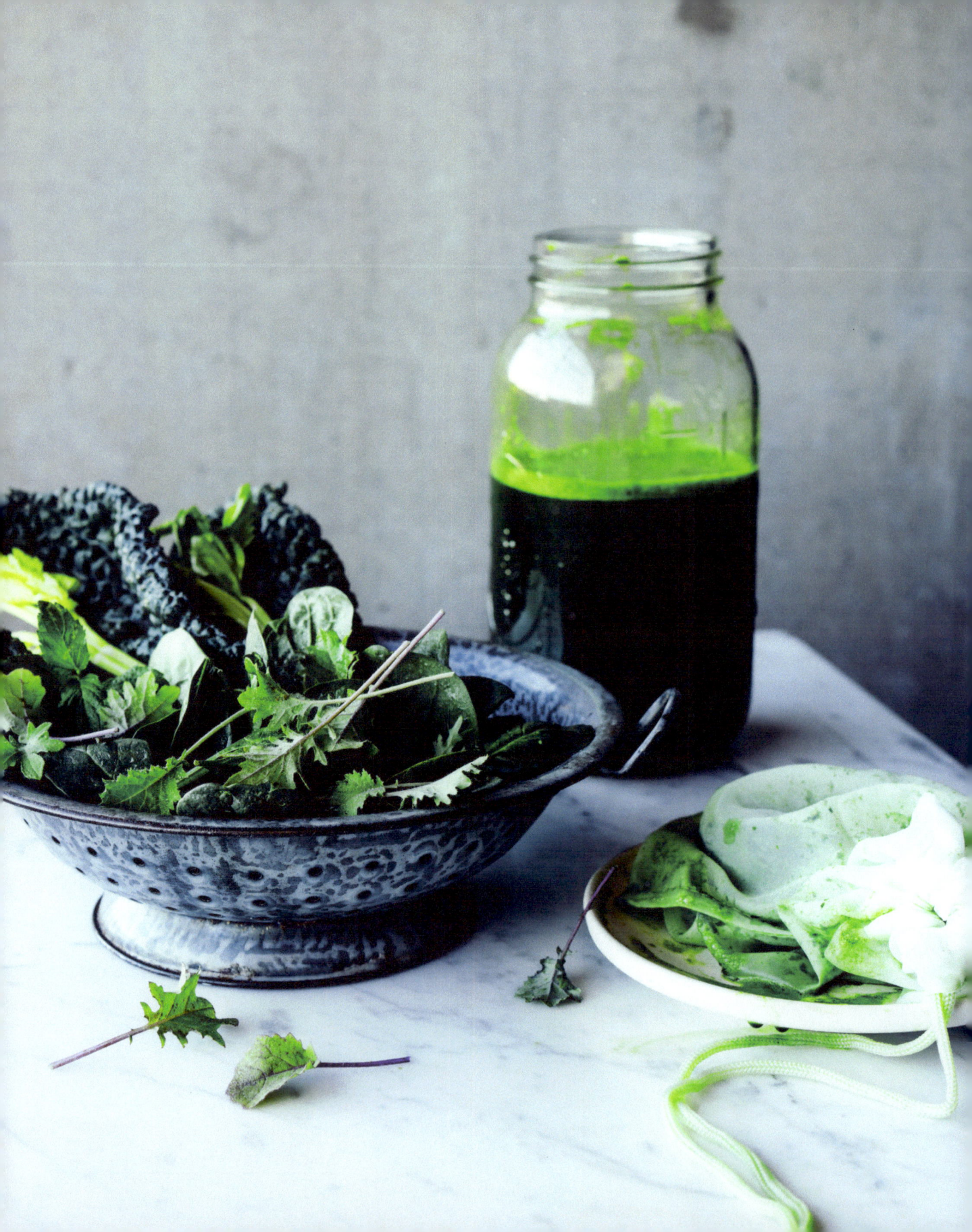

"PRESSED" GREEN JUICE

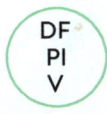

DF
PI
V

Makes 2 servings

½ bunch collard greens

½ bunch kale

2 celery stalks or
1 small cucumber

2 cups filtered water
or coconut water

½ bunch parsley

Handful of baby spinach

Nut-milk strainer bag

1. Chop the collards, kale, and celery into small pieces. Put them in a high-powered blender, add the filtered water, and blend for 30 seconds. Add the parsley and spinach and blend until you have a rich green puree.

2. Pour the puree through the nut strainer placed over a bowl. Strain the juice, using your hands to push all the liquid out from the pulp. (Discard the pulp.)

3. Drink your juice, enjoying all of the amazing benefits!

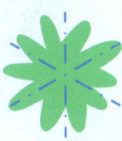

TIP

This juice can be made in advance and kept in the refrigerator for up to 24 hours. Make sure to shake it before drinking, as it will separate. Lightly steaming the greens makes them easier to digest and all of the nutrients more readily available.

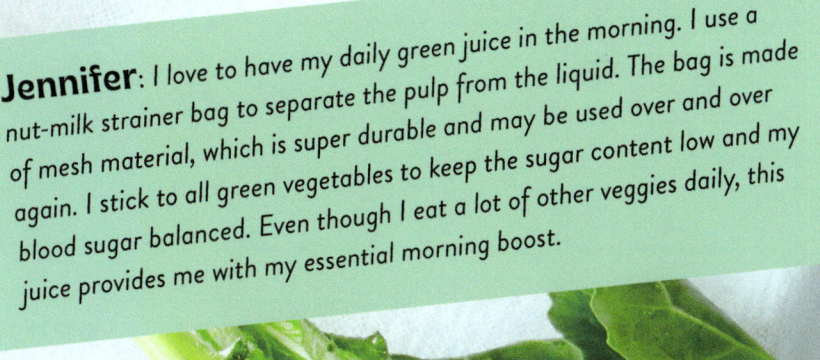

Jennifer: I love to have my daily green juice in the morning. I use a nut-milk strainer bag to separate the pulp from the liquid. The bag is made of mesh material, which is super durable and may be used over and over again. I stick to all green vegetables to keep the sugar content low and my blood sugar balanced. Even though I eat a lot of other veggies daily, this juice provides me with my essential morning boost.

CHERRY ON TOP SMOOTHIE

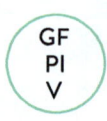

GF
PI
V

Cherries and bananas are great for muscle recovery after a big workout, while the greens and avocado supply an antioxidant boost. This beverage is fun for the whole family!

Makes about two 10-ounce servings

Flesh of ½ avocado (see Tip)

1 banana

1 cup frozen pitted cherries

1 cup chopped greens of your choice (spinach, beet greens, Swiss chard, or kale), lightly steamed (see Tip on page 149)

¼ teaspoon ground cinnamon

2 tablespoons raw cacao powder

1 teaspoon raw honey

1 cup milk of your choice (whole milk, almond milk, or rice milk)

2 cups ice cubes

Place all of the ingredients in a blender and blend for approximately 2 minutes, until well-blended and smooth. Serve immediately.

TIP

We tend to use the avocados that have been in the refrigerator for a day or two for smoothies and open new ones for salads and sauces.

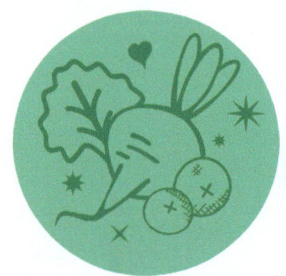

MAGIC MONKEY

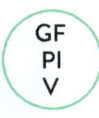

GF PI V

This smoothie has the peanut butter cup flavor that we loved as kids. It is a good-for-you treat that is a powerful energizer post workout or as a midday snack.

Makes about two 10-ounce servings

3 dates

1½ bananas

1½ cups milk of choice (whole milk, almond milk, or rice milk)

2 tablespoons sunflower or almond butter (see Tip)

1 tablespoon raw cacao powder

2 teaspoons raw honey

2 teaspoons spirulina

3 cups ice cubes

Put all of the ingredients in a blender and blend for approximately 2 minutes, until smooth but still thick. Serve immediately.

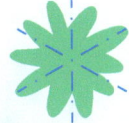

TIP

You can substitute cashew, macadamia, or peanut butter as the nut butter.

Jessica: Raw honey, especially honey that is local to where you live, is a very healing food. It is rich in live enzymes, which are beneficial for digestion, and it is very energizing. I experimented on my child (who loves honey) by giving her 2 teaspoons of raw local honey every morning to build her immune system and to help with the seasonal allergies she typically gets in the springtime. She no longer gets allergies from pollen and her immune health is strong. Having the raw honey every day, which is rich in local pollen, gave her small doses of the pollen so her body became used to it.

DAILY DOSE SMOOTHIE

This vitamin-packed smoothie is a great way to get your daily dose before you even walk out the door. It includes plenty of high-energy foods, rich in antioxidants and protein. Raw eggs are extremely healthful, but it is important to use eggs from a sanitary source: That means choosing free-range, pastured, organic eggs whenever possible to avoid unwanted bacteria. The yolk of the egg has the most vitamins, minerals, and good fats.

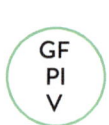

GF
PI
V

*Makes two
10-ounce servings*

2 lightly soft-boiled
free-range eggs boiled
for about 1 minute

2 cups chopped greens
(spinach, beet greens,
Swiss chard, or kale),
lightly steamed (see
Tip on page 149)

1 cup frozen berries
of choice

Flesh of ½ avocado

½ cup milk of choice
(whole milk, almond
milk, or rice milk)

2 cups ice cubes

Combine all of the ingredients in a blender and blend for approximately 2 minutes, until smooth but still thick. Serve immediately.

TIP

We believe in using just the yolks in the smoothie because they are more easily digested, much higher in nutritional value than the whites and are much lower in possible allergens.

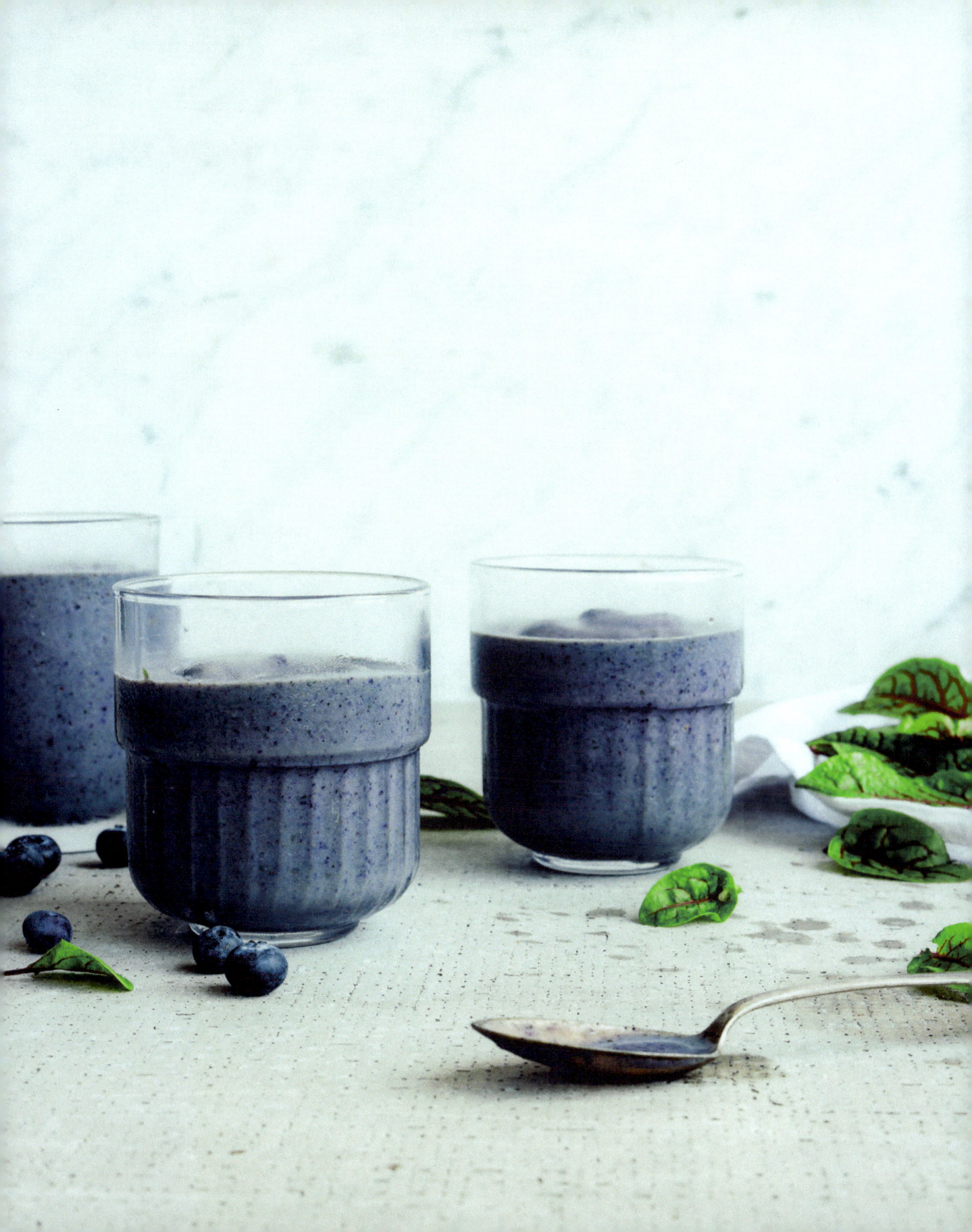

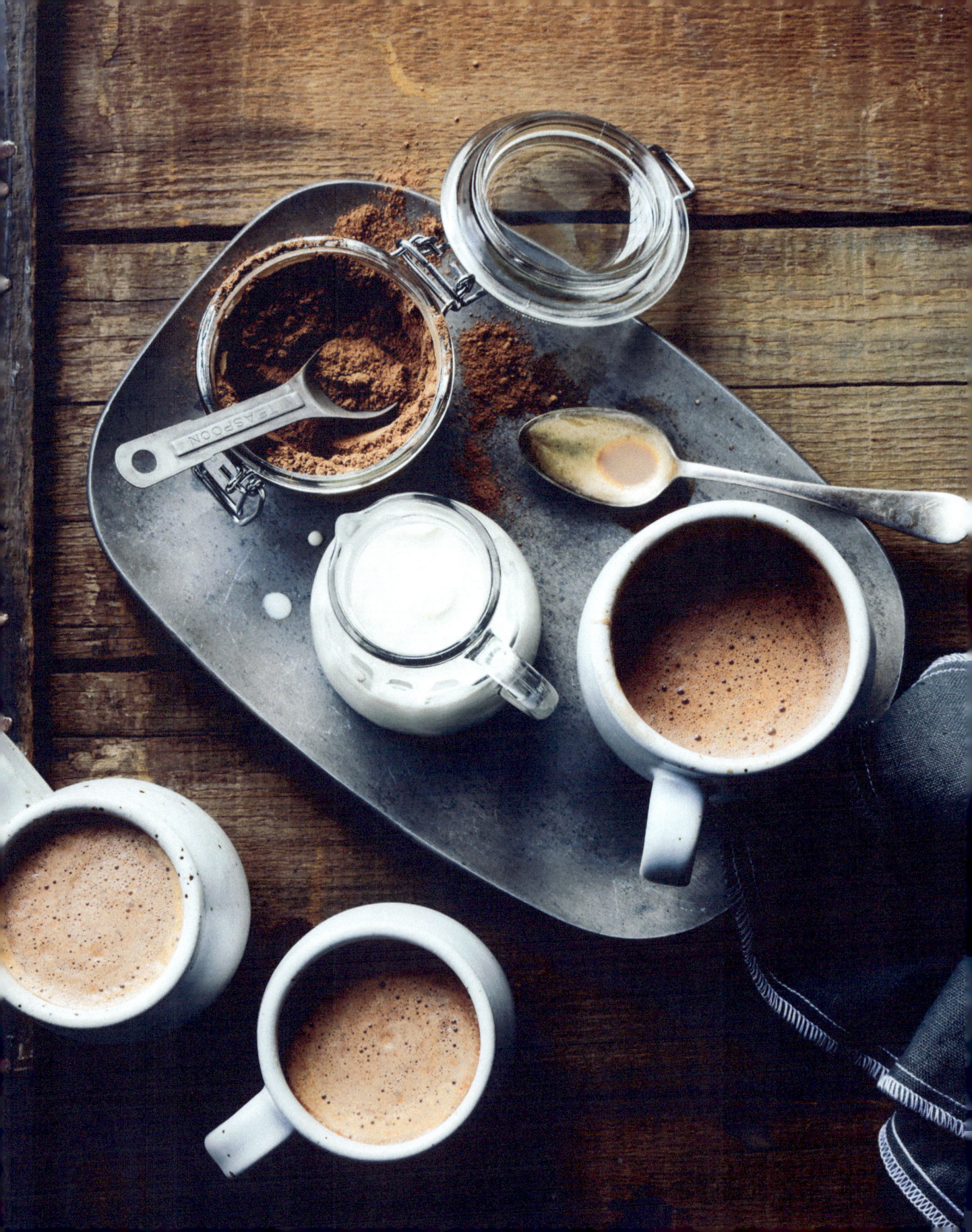

ROOT TO RISE COFFEE

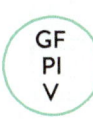

**GF
PI
V**

Putting fat such as ghee and coconut milk or cream into your coffee helps to metabolize the caffeine more slowly, keeping you from getting jittery and then crashing. It also assists in brain function and boosts energy. Enjoy the buzzzzzzz.

*Makes about two
10-ounce mugs*

2 cups freshly
brewed coffee

½ cup full-fat canned
coconut milk or
grass-fed cream

2 heaping table-
spoons raw cacao

2 tablespoons
grass-fed ghee

1. Add all of the ingredients to the blender and blend, starting on low and gradually increasing to high, for a total of about 30 seconds.

2. Serve hot and frothy from the blender.

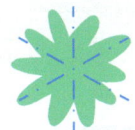

TIP

This coffee is wonderful as is, but it's also delicious served with about ½ tablespoon of honey, maple syrup, or your favorite natural sweetener.

FAT IS FABULOUS

We are big BIG advocates for good fats. It is one of the foundational building blocks in our diets. It helps maintain our energy and keeps our brainpower in tiptop shape. Healthy fats help build cell walls and make it easier for nutrients to get in to our system. Our brains are made up of about 60% fat, so eating good fats helps with brain function, too. Fats also help regulate blood sugar and stabilize our metabolisms so we feel satiated and avoid that constant tug to run to the fridge or pantry for high-carb, high-salt, or sugary snacks.

When we say good fats, we mean luscious, nourishing, cell-building, heart-healthy fats like olive oil and coconut oil, not processed ones like corn, soy, canola, or safflower fats. Including healthy fats in your diet can actually help you shed weight and keep you feeling energized and alert. It is the good stuff. And to really reap the benefits of the good stuff, it is also important to simultaneously cut down on processed sugars and refined carbs.

Below we provide an overview of our favorite fats, which we use throughout the book, along with best uses for each. More stable fats with higher smoke temperatures are better for cooking, while some of the others are best used in vinaigrettes and to drizzle on finished dishes for added flavor and nutritional value. Smoke temperature is the point at which an oil literally starts to smoke when overheated. As it smokes, it loses its nutritional value and can even release toxins; it also can impart a burnt or "off" flavor to the food you are preparing.

Extra-virgin olive oil: EVOO is an excellent oil for vinaigrettes, and as a finishing oil. You can cook with extra-virgin olive oil, too, as it is more stable than a lot of other oils. However, it does start to lose valuable nutritional elements at higher temperatures, so choose another fat for hightemperature cooking. EVOO is high in antioxidants and can help reduce inflammation in the body.

Coconut oil: This is a healthy unsaturated fat to use when roasting, sautéing, frying, and baking. Unrefined coconut oil is better to use than refined, because it is in its "pure" form, meaning it has more nutritional value and is not processed in any way. It is also more stable at higher temperatures. Keep in mind that it does have more of a coconut flavor than refined versions. Coconut oil can aid in weight loss, boost the immune system, assist with proper digestion, and regulate the metabolism.

Toasted and untoasted sesame oil: These are great oils for finishing sauces, dressings, and sautéing. Untoasted sesame oil is a good choice for stir-fries and sautés, while toasted sesame oil is better for drizzling, as it has a strong flavor and thus should be used sparingly. These oils are very high in linoleic acid, which is one of the two essential fatty acids that our bodies cannot produce. This fatty acid is necessary for healthy blood, arteries, and nerves. It can also help our skin and other tissues stay youthful by preventing dryness.

Ghee/Clarified Butter: Ghee is an excellent option when frying, sautéing, roasting, and baking. Ghee is butter with the milk solids removed. This is done to enhance the butter flavor and makes it more stable for cooking over heat. It also enhances the health benefits. Ghee can help heal your digestive tract, balance your cholesterol levels, and increase your energy level. It is a staple in Ayurvedic and Indian cooking. We love to make our own (for recipe, see page 24).

"Life is Change. Change is Life. Nothing stays the same. Eventually everything we hold on to must be let go. Trust and acceptance are our guides and love is the way."

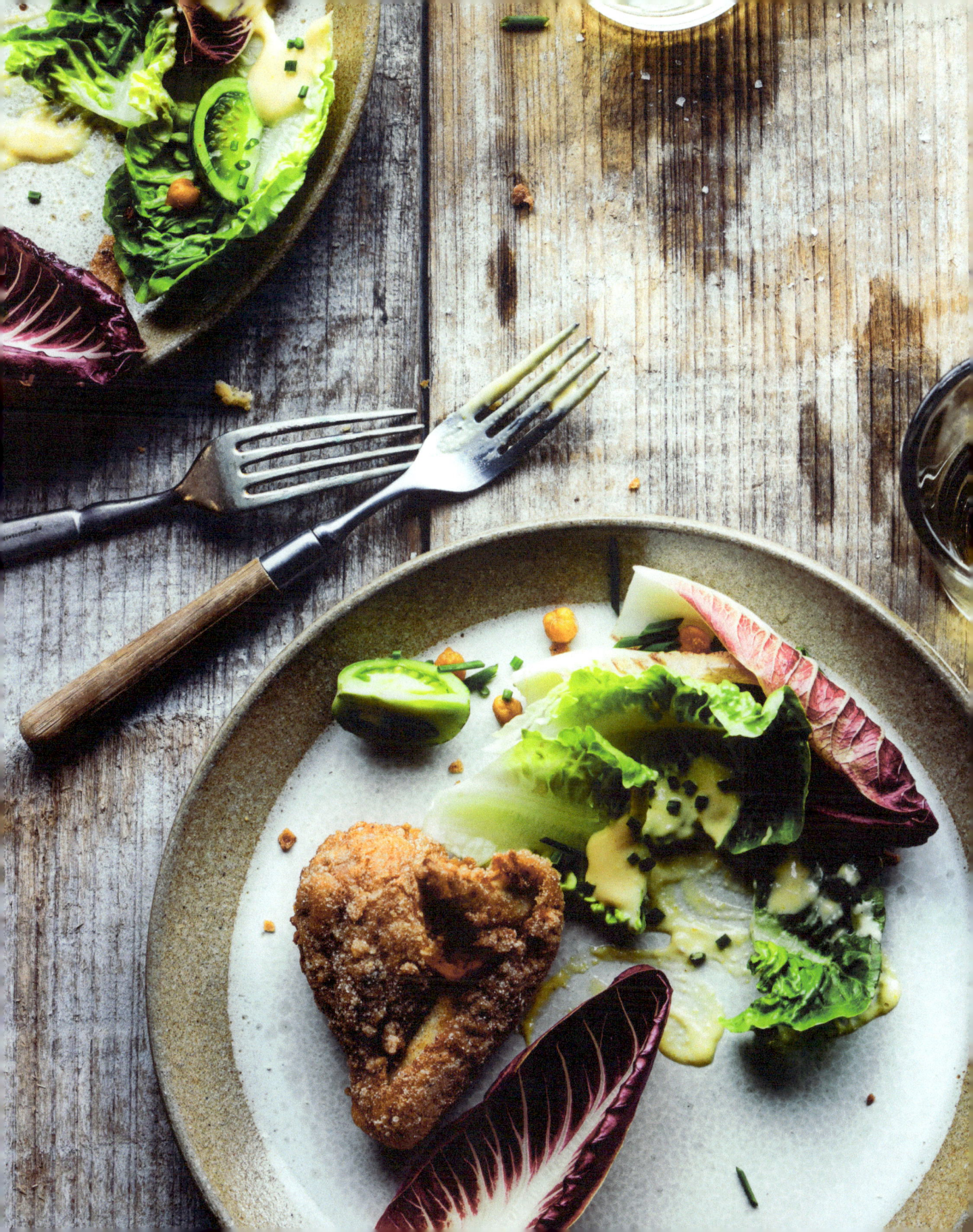

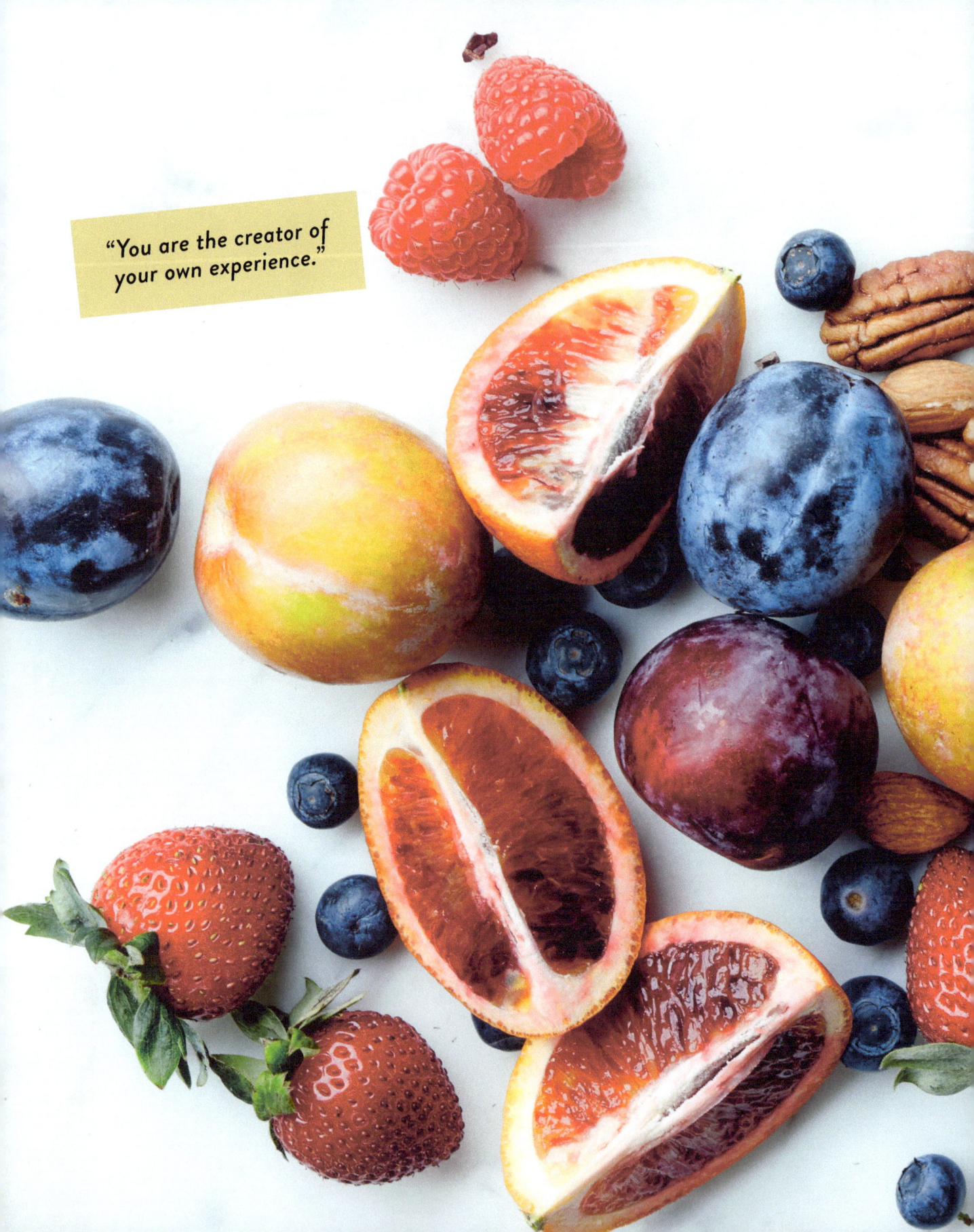

"You are the creator of your own experience."

SWEETS & TREATS

We'd be hard-pressed to find someone who is not a sweets person. The real challenge is that oftentimes sweets are processed and refined, which makes them unhealthy. But if you use nutrient-rich whole food ingredients like raw cacao, almond flour, coconut oil, pumpkin puree, and raw honey, sweets can be good for you. Our recipes are not only delicious but nutritious and they will satisfy. Our theory is to indulge, not deprive! You can have it all, even when it comes to dessert.

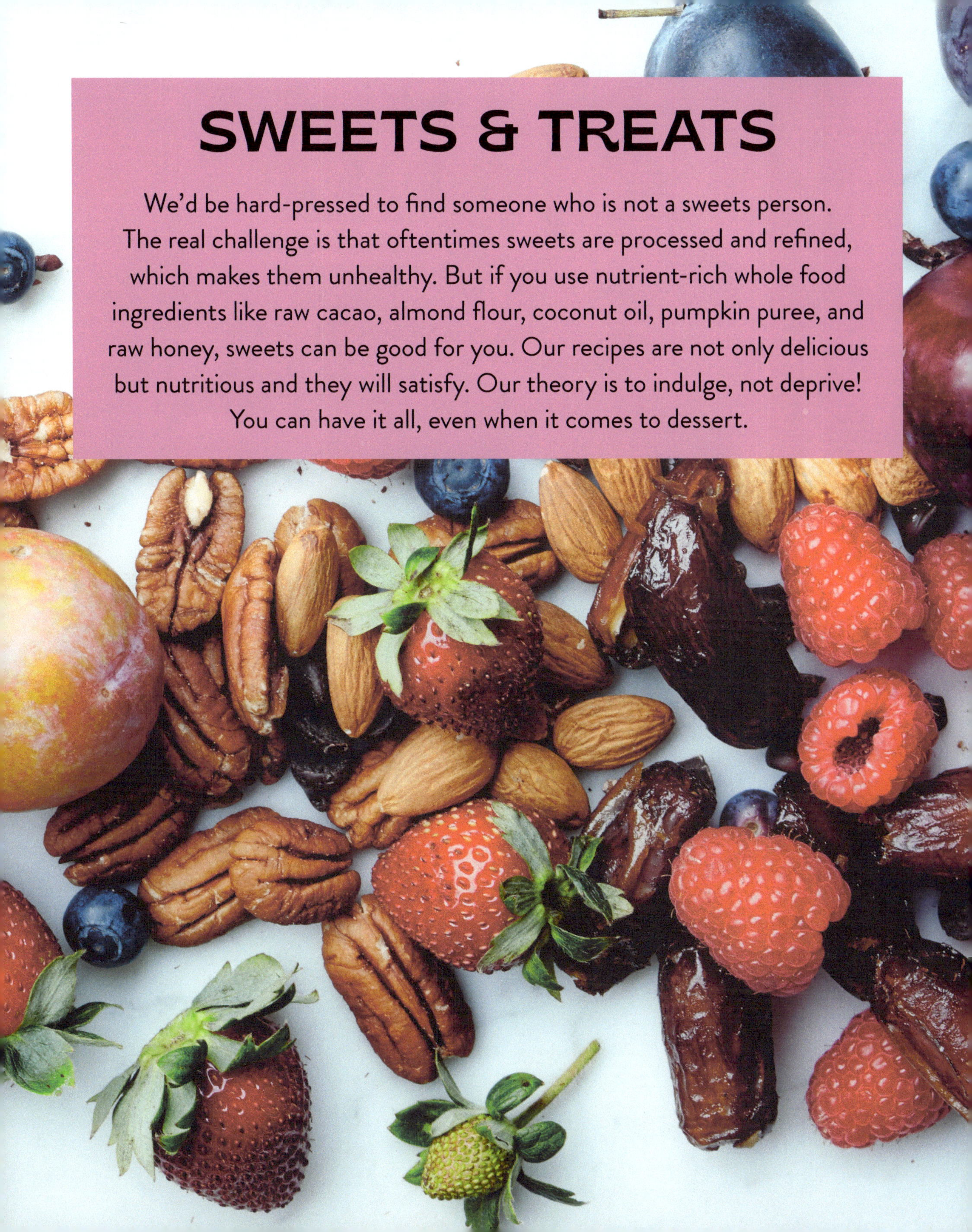

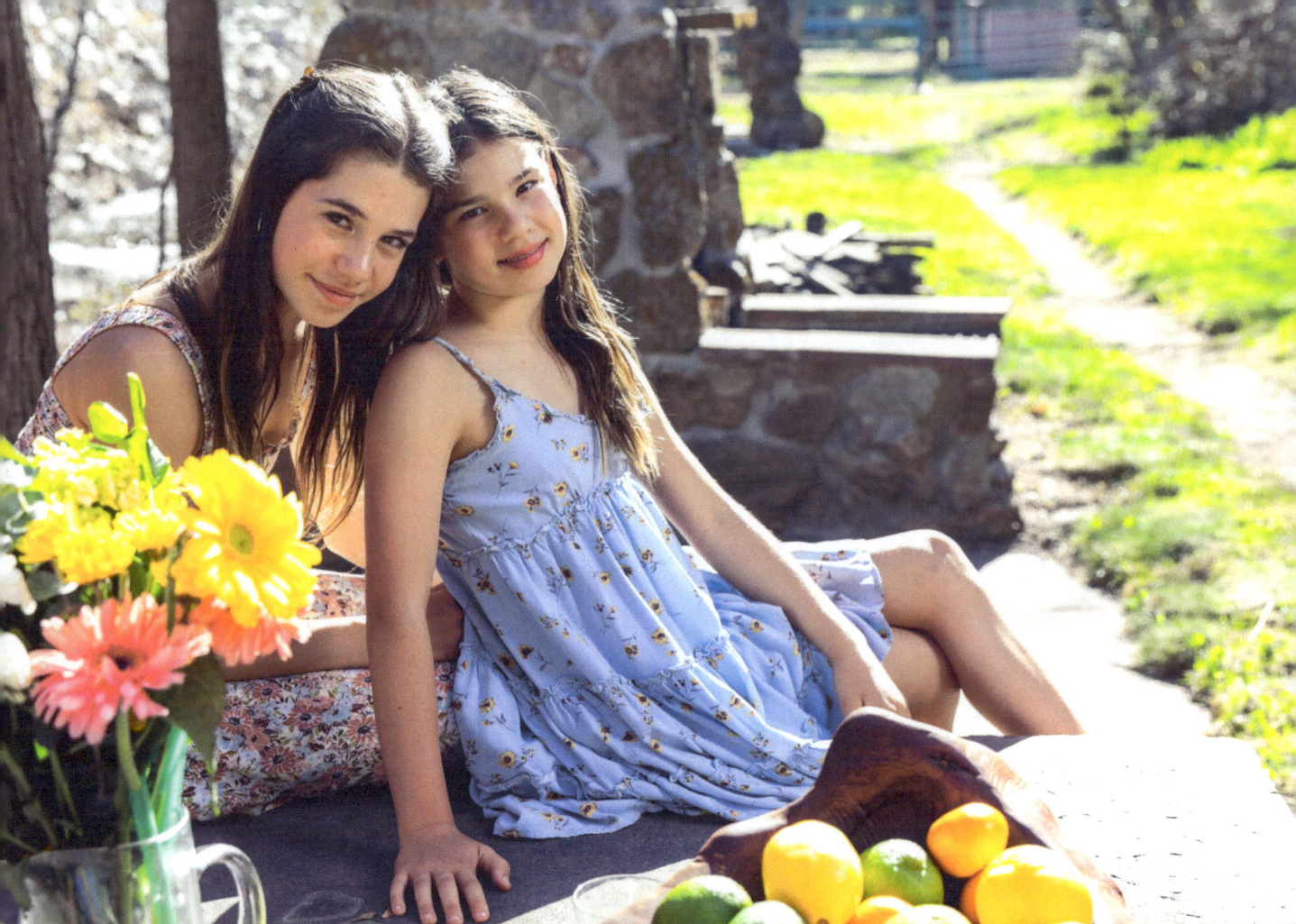

Jessica: *I have thought a lot about how to help my kids have a healthy relationship to sweets since, like all kids, they are hard-wired to love them. I want my kids to enjoy sweets and indulge occasionally, but not feel like that is all they want or crave. One of the ways I attempt to forge this healthy relationship is to have them start the day with something savory as opposed to sweet. I have noticed that on days when I give them a sweet breakfast, they crave more sweets throughout the day. I also started them early in their lives on things like raw sauerkrauts, broths, grass-fed ground meats, pastured eggs, ghee, and wholesome vegetables. (I'm telling you start them young and it is possible!)*

Another one of my goals is to not to offer sweets to them at home unless it's a healthy kind of sweet such as our homemade ice pops or jello (pages 164 and 167). They will be offered plenty of sugary treats while they are out in the world, so I let them get it outside the home. I also decided not to reward my kids with sweets because it can send a message that sweets are fun and good while other foods are not. I believe we as parents have a huge influence on how our kids relate to sweets and food in general. It is a good reminder for me to check in on my own relationship with food

THE SKINNY ON SWEETS

We all have a relationship with sweets. For some of us, they feel like a naughty indulgence. We may even feel dependent on them for happiness or satisfaction, and want more as soon as the sugar rush is gone.

Sweets are tricky that way. Sugar is hidden in many processed foods, which is just one more reason why we are big advocates for a whole-food lifestyle. It acts like a drug and can be addictive, releasing dopamine in the body to give us a sugar high, and then when it wears off, sending us into withdrawal and wanting more. Most of us have experienced this dynamic on some level and it becomes draining pretty quickly. Excess sugar depletes our nervous system and immune system, increases inflammation in the body, and contributes to weight gain by building resistance to certain hormones that regulate the metabolism.

Cutting out processed sugars will absolutely single-handedly improve your health. But we get it, sweets are feel-good food for many of us, so we are here to talk to you about how to satisfy that sweet tooth in a way that actually satiates your body. You can create a relationship with sweets that is satisfying, good for you, and empowering. Here are a few of our favorite alternative sweeteners.

Local raw honey has not been heat-treated or pro-cessed so all of the powerful enzymes, vitamins, and minerals are intact. It has antibacterial properties and can help strengthen the immune system. It can also be great for allergies: If taken before the allergy season starts, local honey can build up immunities to certain pollens because the honey contains small amounts of pollen from the local environment.

Coconut sugar is made from the sap of the coconut palm that has been extracted, boiled, dehydrated, and granulated. It has a rich flavor almost like brown sugar.

Pure maple syrup contains important antioxidants and minerals. The darker and richer in color and flavor, the more nutritional value it has. Make sure to choose pure maple syrup or it will most likely have refined sugar added. Each of these sweeteners metabolize in your system more slowly and are more stabilizing than processed sugars. But even so, it is still sensible to use them in moderation because eating sweets—even these healthier alternatives—can sometimes make you crave more sweets.

When you are experiencing a craving for a sweet treat, here are a few quick snacks that will give you imme-diate satisfaction without making your blood sugar go crazy:

Frozen grapes: Throw a bag of grapes in the freezer to munch on when you want a sweet snack. They have tons of antioxidants and help with digestion and hydration, too.

Watermelon with coconut cream: You know the cream that sits at the top of a can of coconut milk? We like to skim it off the top and mix it with some watermelon or berries for a delicious treat. To make it separate more easily, refrigerate a can of coconut milk—the cream will rise to the top.

A bowl of frozen berries topped with your favorite milk: The frozen berries may cause the milk to get slushy (depending on the milk you choose), but slushy or not, grab a spoon and satisfy that sweet tooth.

Warm milk or boiled water with raw cacao powder: When you want a cup of hot chocolate, try this combination instead and, if you so desire, add a touch of one of the alternative sweeteners listed above or a drop of peppermint oil or both. This drink is warming and will help quench your thirst for chocolate. (If you want to avoid any caffeine stimulation, substitute carob powder for the raw cacao.)

Slices of apple or banana with unsweetened almond or other nut butter and local raw honey: This combi-nation gives you energy-producing protein on top of quelling your sugar craving.

A few squares of dark chocolate: It contains a ton of antioxidants and is a great quick fix. Make sure to look for a cacao content of 70 percent or higher since this will ensure lower sugar and more antioxidants. To up the ante, smear on some nut butter.

RAW CHEESECAKE WITH CHERRY SAUCE

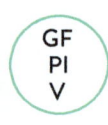

GF
PI
V

We have vivid memories of Mom making cheesecake throughout our child-hood. She always let us put the graham crackers in a bag and take turns with the rolling pin to crumble the crackers for the crust. She would top this cake with a sweet cherry sauce that was unforgettable. This is a raw version of our favorite dessert made by Mom.

*Makes one
9-inch cake*

CRUST:

1 cup raw almonds

½ cup pitted dates
(approximately 5 or 6
dates, preferably Medjool)

½ cup raw coconut flakes

½ teaspoon vanilla
extract (to make your
own, see opposite)

1 small pinch sea salt

FILLING:

3 cups raw cashews,
soaked in warm water
for at least 2 hours

¾ cup fresh lemon juice
(from about 3 lemons)

½ cup plus 1 table-
spoon raw honey

¾ cup coconut oil

1 tablespoon vanilla
extract (to make your
own, see opposite)

1 small pinch sea salt

Fresh Cherry Sauce
(recipe opposite)

1. Make the crust: Put the almonds in a food processor and run until the almonds are finely ground. Add the dates, coconut flakes, vanilla, and salt and process until thoroughly combined. The mixture should stick between your fingers when squeezed. Remove from the food processor and form into a ball.

2. Put the ball of dough in an ungreased 9-inch springform pan or pie pan (see Tip). Press the ball of dough into the prepared pan, working it up the sides of the pan, until the crust is ½-inch thick throughout and covers the bottom and sides of the pan evenly.

3. Make the filling: Rinse and drain the cashews. Transfer to a clean food processor, add the lemon juice, honey, coconut oil, and salt. Puree until the filling is silky smooth, approximately 90 seconds.

4. Pour the filling into the crust, smoothing the top with a spatula. Put the cheesecake in the freezer for at least 1 hour to set. (The cheesecake can be made up to 3 days ahead.)

5. If you're using a springform pan, remove the sides of the pan before serving. Top the whole cheesecake or slices of the cake with the cherry sauce.

TIP

We find this recipe works best in a springform pan, but it can be made in a regular pie pan as well. You may have a little bit of extra cashew filling if using a pie pan. We love drizzling this over fresh fruit, fruit salad, or toast.

FRESH CHERRY SAUCE

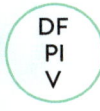

**DF
PI
V**

Makes about 1 cup

1½ cups fresh or frozen
pitted cherries

2 tablespoons coconut oil

2 teaspoons maple syrup

1. In a blender, combine 1 cup of the cherries with the coconut oil and maple syrup and blend until smooth. (Add a touch of water to keep things moving if necessary, but use as little as possible; the sauce should be thick.)

2. Chop the remaining ½ cup cherries and put them into a small mixing bowl.

3. Stir the cherry puree into the chopped cherries. Chill for at least 10 minutes before serving. The sauce can be made up to 3 days ahead and refrigerated in an airtight container.

GLUTEN-FREE VANILLA EXTRACT

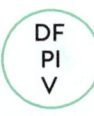

**DF
PI
V**

Makes 3 cups

9 vanilla beans

1 (750-ml) bottle of
gluten-free vodka, such
as potato or grape vodka

1. Using a sharp paring knife, cut each vanilla bean lengthwise in half, leaving an inch at one end connected. Add the vanilla beans directly to the bottle of vodka and replace the cap tightly.

2. Store in a dark, cool place for 3 to 4 months, giving the bottle a shake every once in a while.

3. After this time period, your vanilla extract is ready for use. No need to strain out the vanilla beans. The extract will last for years in your pantry.

TIP

Gluten-free vanilla extract is hard to find in stores and can be expensive. This may seem like a lot of vanilla extract, but it has a long shelf life and is a quick, easy, and less expensive way to make it yourself. If you want to make less, use 3 vanilla beans per cup of vodka. Store in a glass bottle with a tight-fitting lid.

MY KID'S FAVORITE POPS

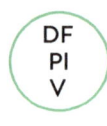

DF
PI
V

Makes six 4-ounce pops or four 6-ounce pops

1½ cups fresh or frozen organic strawberries or blueberries or a combination

2 tablespoons raw honey

1½ cups plain yogurt or full-fat canned coconut milk

½ tablespoon vanilla extract (to make your own, see page 163)

1. Puree the berries in a high-powered blender or food processor. Add 1 tablespoon of the honey to the berry puree and blend until combined.

2. In a small bowl, stir together the yogurt, vanilla extract, and remaining tablespoon of honey until combined thoroughly.

3. Pour 1 to 2 tablespoons of the berry puree into each pop mold. Spoon in 1 to 2 tablespoons of the yogurt mixture on top. Alternate between the berry puree and yogurt mixture for a layered effect until the molds are full.

4. Freeze the pops for at least 6 hours before serving (see Tip). They will keep in the freezer for at least 2 months.

TIP

Your ice pops should be completely frozen before serving. To help release the frozen pops from their molds, run the bottom of the molds under warm water for about 30 seconds.

Jessica: These pops are a staple in our freezer year-round. They are simple, delicious, and I like that this recipe has so few ingredients, which makes it easy on the body, as opposed to store-bought brands that usually contain many different ingredients and preservatives.

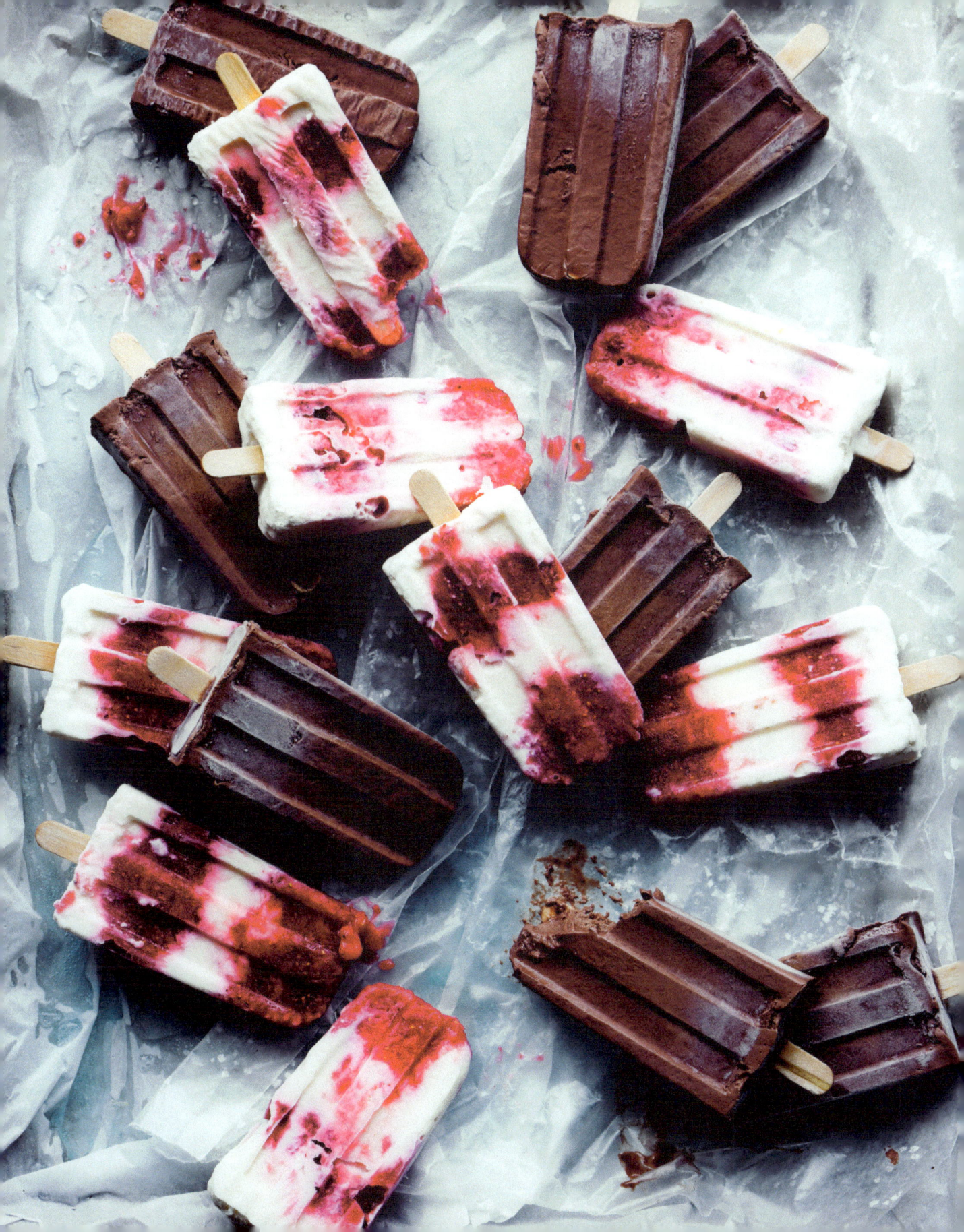

FROZEN FUDGE POPS

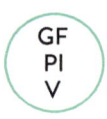

GF
PI
V

Fudge pops at the store are usually loaded with refined sugar and preservatives. This is our good-for-you version. This treat incorporates many healing foods—each ingredient is powerful in its own right—while satisfying your chocolate craving on a hot day.

Makes six 4-ounce pops or four 6-ounce pops

2 (14-ounce) cans full-fat coconut milk

1½ teaspoons vanilla extract (to make your own, see page 163)

3½ tablespoons raw honey

½ cup raw cacao powder (or carob powder if you would like a caffeine-free alternative)

1½ tablespoons grass-fed unflavored gelatin powder

1. In a small saucepan on medium heat, warm the coconut milk until nearly boiling. Whisk in the vanilla and honey. Reduce the heat to a simmer. Whisk in the cacao powder until thoroughly combined. Turn the burner off.

2. Sprinkle the gelatin over the surface of the coconut milk mixture. Let it sit for 3 to 4 minutes to allow it to activate, then whisk the gelatin into the milk mixture until all the lumps are gone. Remove the pan from the stovetop and allow it to cool for 20 to 30 minutes.

3. Pour the cooled coconut milk mixture into the ice pop molds (see Tip), dividing it evenly. Freeze the pops completely before serving. They will be ready in 6 to 8 hours.

TIP

If you don't have ice pop molds, small paper cups can be used instead. Fill the cups an inch or two from the top of the cup of the cooled coconut milk mixture and let it freeze long enough to hold the pop sticks upright, about 45 minutes. Insert the sticks, fill the cups completely, and return to the freezer. When fully frozen, peel away the paper from the pops and enjoy.

GOOD FOR YOU JELLO

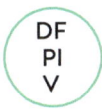

DF
PI
V

*Makes one
8-inch pan*

1½ tablespoons grass-fed
unflavored gelatin powder

½ cup cool water

½ cup hot (almost
boiling) water

1½ cups white grape juice

½ cup cranberry
juice (see Tip)

1 cup sliced strawberries

1. Put the gelatin in a large bowl. Add the cool water and whisk vigorously until the gelatin thickens. Add the hot water and stir to mix; the mixture will thin out a bit. Add the grape and cranberry juices and mix well.

2. Put the strawberries in an 8-inch glass pan (a square baking dish or a pie plate work well). Pour the gelatin mixture over the berries and stir gently.

3. Cover the pan with plastic wrap and put it in the fridge until firm, at least 3 hours or overnight.

4. Cut into cubes, scoop it with a melon baller, or use cookie cutters to make cute shapes for serving.

TIP

You can definitely play with the types of juices used in this recipe. I have, on occasion, even used freshly juiced juices.

Jessica: My daughter's friend always says this tastes like gummy bears. Little does she know the nutrients I sneak in! Grass-fed gelatin is a surprising superfood. Gelatin works from the inside out to help strengthen hair and nails, give skin a healthy glow, as well as improving the health of joints, ligaments, and tendons.

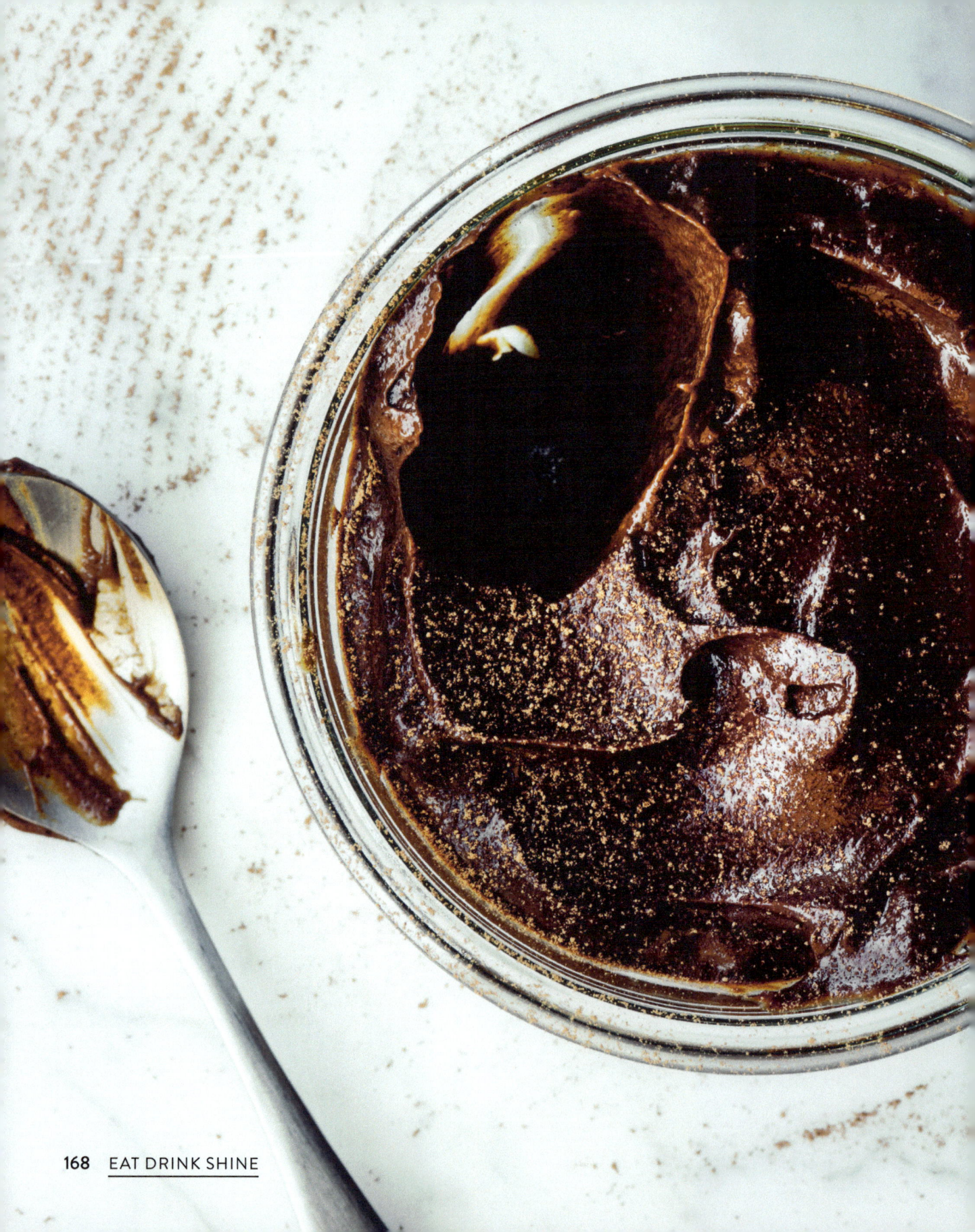

BANANA CHOCOLATE MOUSSE

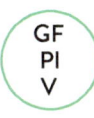

GF
PI
V

Carob and raw cacao can be used interchangeably in this recipe. Carob is a chocolate alternative, for people who don't do caffeine or stimulants—or don't want caffeine before bed. It is a legume that doesn't taste exactly like chocolate but has a similar flavor. Raw cacao is chocolate in its purest form and it is Paleo friendly. This mousse is great topped with berries, nuts, coconut flakes, etc. Kids love this healthy dessert!

Makes about 4 cups; serves 4 to 6

10 dates, pitted and soaked in water for 2 to 3 hours

1 ripe banana, peeled and roughly sliced

3 ripe avocados, pitted, flesh scooped out of shells

½ cup maple syrup

¼ cup raw honey (local if possible)

½ cup raw cacao powder or carob powder

2 teaspoon vanilla extract (to make your own, see page 163)

Put the drained dates in a food processor and process for 1 minute. (The dates will form a ball. This is fine.) Add the banana and avocados and process for another minute. Add the maple syrup, honey, cacao, and vanilla and process for 1 minute more. Chill the mousse in the refrigerator for at least an hour before serving. Store in an airtight container; it will keep in the refrigerator for up to 3 days.

TIP

This can also be used as a healthy vegan chocolate frosting or whipped cream for cakes, cupcakes, and ice cream.

RAW CHOCOLATE TRUFFLES

We are lucky enough to enjoy these truffles almost daily. They are always on the menu at the restaurant and they are our sweet treat after meals. It is fun to experiment with flavors—we sometimes even add medicinal herbs and spices. These are very satisfying because even though a single truffle makes just a small dessert, they have the perfect amount of sweetness to satisfy any sweet tooth.

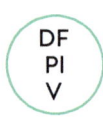

DF
PI
V

Makes 10 truffles
1 cup whole raw almonds
¼ cup coconut oil
¼ cup raw honey
¾ cup cacao powder
2 teaspoons sea salt

1. Put the almonds in a food processor and blend until they almost form a butter, about 2 to 3 minutes. Transfer to a large bowl.

2. Warm the coconut oil to a pourable consistency. Pour the oil into the ground almonds, add the honey, cacao, and salt, and mix well.

3. Spread the truffle mixture into a small baking pan or food-storage container, cover with plastic wrap, and put in the refrigerator to cool until it hardens, at least 6 hours or overnight.

4. Using a tablespoon or melon baller, scoop about 2 tablespoons of the truffle mixture at a time and roll it with your hands into small balls. Arrange the truffles on a platter and serve immediately.

TIP

There are many variations on these truffles you can make. For example, for our Cherry Vanilla Truffles, we add 2 tablespoons chopped dried cherries and 2 teaspoons vanilla extract to the truffle base. Let your imagination and your tastebuds be your guide.

RAW CHOCOLATE CHIP COOKIE DOUGH

One of our earliest cooking memories is of the three of us climbing atop chairs to reach the counter to help our mom make chocolate chip cookies. The combination of brown sugar, butter, and vanilla with chocolate chips made licking the bowl and spoon so unbelievably heavenly—though there is nothing that causes ear-piercing screaming like trying to share two batter-filled beaters between three little girls. And we definitely snuck some dough while mom wasn't looking, so that experience very often ended in a tummy ache! This is our version that is reminiscent of that experience, but much easier on the belly. Enjoy the dough on its own with a spoon or as a spread on fruit such as apples, bananas, and pears.

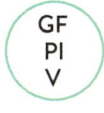

GF
PI
V

Makes 2 cups
1 cup raw tahini (sesame seed paste)

¼ cup plus 3 tablespoons raw honey

3 tablespoons coconut oil

1 teaspoon vanilla extract (to make your own, see page 163)

Tiny pinch of sea salt

¼ cup cacao or carob chips

Put the tahini, honey, coconut oil, vanilla, and salt in a food processor and process for 1 minute. Pour the "batter" into a small bowl and stir in the chips. Cover and refrigerate for up to 5 days.

TIP

To make a healthier version of cookie dough ice cream, add this to softened homemade vanilla ice cream, right out of the ice cream maker.

Jill: Can't stop, won't stop. This one is dangerously delicious AND oh so good for you, so dig in! The consistency varies depending on the brand of tahini you use. I like thicker tahini, but my husband likes it with thinner, so find which one floats your boat.

CHOCOLATE CHIP PALEO COOKIES

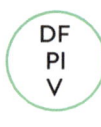

DF
PI
V

Makes 20 cookies

2½ cups almond flour

½ teaspoon sea salt

½ teaspoon baking soda

½ cup coconut oil, melted, plus more for greasing

½ cup maple syrup

2 teaspoons vanilla extract (to make your own, see page 163)

1 cup dark chocolate chips

1. Mix together the almond flour, salt, and baking soda in a large bowl.

2. Blend together the coconut oil, maple syrup, and vanilla in a small bowl.

3. Pour the wet ingredients into the dry ingredients and mix together well. Stir in the chocolate chips and let the dough chill for at least 1 hour in the refrigerator (see Tip).

4. When you're ready to bake the cookies, preheat the oven to 350°F. Line a baking sheet with parchment paper or grease it with coconut oil.

5. Scoop approximately 8 balls of dough, each about 1 tablespoon in size, onto the prepared baking sheet. (Do not crowd the pan.) Bake for approximately 10 minutes, until lightly golden, and then transfer the cookies to a cooling rack. Repeat with the remaining cookie dough.

6. Serve warm or store in an airtight container for up to 5 days.

TIP

You can also make the dough ahead of time and freeze it, wrapped in a double layer of plastic. Thaw it in the refrigerator overnight before baking.

Jill: My husband Steve is a Shine cookie monster and master and I love when he starts whipping these up after dinner. My nieces love them, house guests love them, and I love them. A total crowd pleaser and simple as all get out. They have excellent flavor and texture, plus the almond flour makes them high in protein. People who can't eat grains, eggs or dairy always go nuts over how good these are.

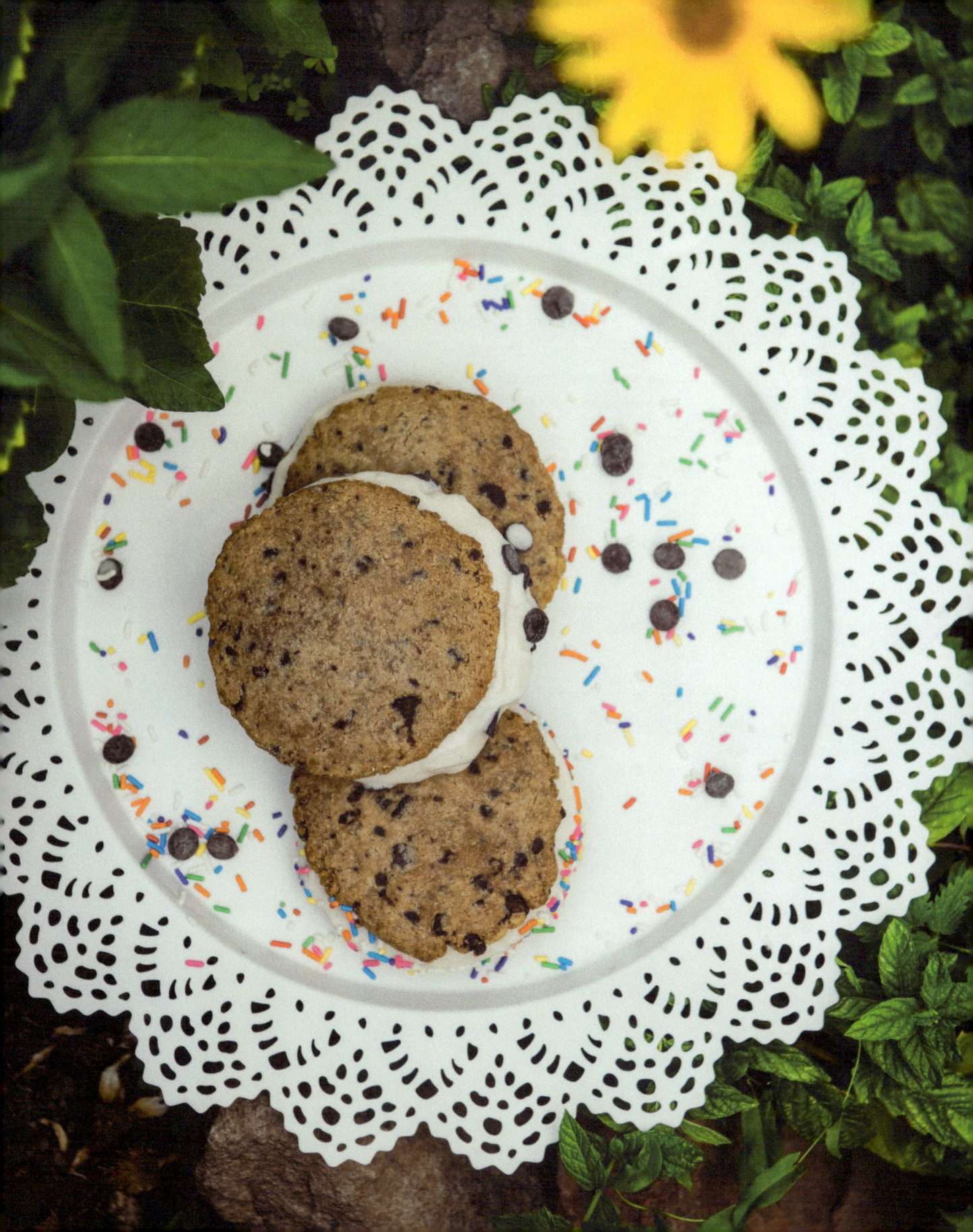

GRAIN-FREE BANANA BREAD

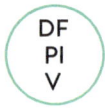

DF
PI
V

*Makes one
9 x 5-inch loaf*

1 tablespoon coconut oil,
plus more for greasing

1 cup smooth
almond butter

2 ripe bananas,
mashed well

¼ cup maple syrup

2 large eggs, whisked

3 tablespoons
coconut flour

2 teaspoons ground
cinnamon

½ teaspoon ground
nutmeg

½ teaspoon baking soda

½ teaspoon baking powder

pinch of sea salt

1. Preheat the oven to 350°F. Grease the loaf pan with coconut oil (see Tip).

2. In a large bowl, mix together well the almond butter, banana, maple syrup, coconut oil, and eggs.

3. In a small bowl, mix together the flour, cinnamon, nutmeg, baking soda and powder, and the salt.

4. Add the dry ingredients to the wet and mix until combined. (It is okay to have some banana chunks.)

5. Pour the batter into the prepared loaf pan and bake for 35 to 40 minutes, until a toothpick or sharp knife inserted into the middle of the loaf comes out clean.

6. Cool the loaf in the pan for about 30 minutes before removing from the pan and slicing and serving. Wrapped in plastic, leftovers will keep for up to 3 days.

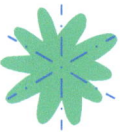

TIP

If you don't have the right size loaf pan, you can use a bigger one and do a shorter baking time. Do not use a smaller loaf pan because ingredients may rise and go over the sides, creating a big mess! This recipe can also be made in a 9 x 9-inch brownie pan, but reduce the cooking time to 30–35 minutes.

Jessica: This is a great grain-free snack or accompaniment to breakfast. My daughter loves when I pack it as a treat with her lunch. We like it smothered with ghee and local raw honey.

DECADENT GRAIN-FREE BEET BROWNIES

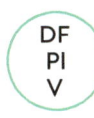

DF
PI
V

Serves about 6

2 medium beets (to make ½ cup beet puree)

1 tablespoon extra-virgin olive oil

2 tablespoons water or apple juice

2 tablespoons coconut oil, plus 1 tablespoon for greasing the pan

¾ cup raw cacao powder

½ cup almond meal

½ cup almond butter

⅓ cup honey

¼ cup high quality maple syrup

1 tablespoon vanilla extract (to make your own, see page 163)

1 teaspoon baking powder

pinch of sea salt

1. Preheat the oven to 375°F.

2. Cut of a sliver on both ends of the beets to remove the root and the stem then scrub the beets to remove any dirt. Put the beets in a small pan (about 8x8) and add 1 cup water and a drizzle of olive oil. Then cover with a piece of foil. Cook the beets for about 45 minutes until they are pierced easily with a sharp knife. Lower oven temperature to 325°F.

3. Let the beets cool and then remove the skins with a paper towel or hand towel. It should come off easily. Roughly chop the beets and put them in a food processor with just a bit of water or apple juice (about 2 tablespoons) to make a puree. Measure out ½ cup of beet puree for the brownies (see Tip).

4. Melt 2 tablespoons of the coconut oil. Mix together all ingredients including the beets and the melted coconut oil in a bowl with a spoon. Mix well until everything is fully incorporated.

5. Grease an 8 x 8-inch pan with the remaining 1 tablespoon of coconut oil. Pour the brownie mixture into the pan and bake uncovered at 325°F for about 45 minutes. To check for doneness, insert a sharp knife or tooth pick into the center. It should come out mostly clean.

6. Let cool for 20 minutes and Enjoy! This stays fresh for about 5 days in the fridge.

TIP

If you have more than 4 beets in the bunch and want to roast them all, roasted beets are excellent sliced and tossed in red wine vinegar or orange juice. Serve them hot or cold in salads or as a side.

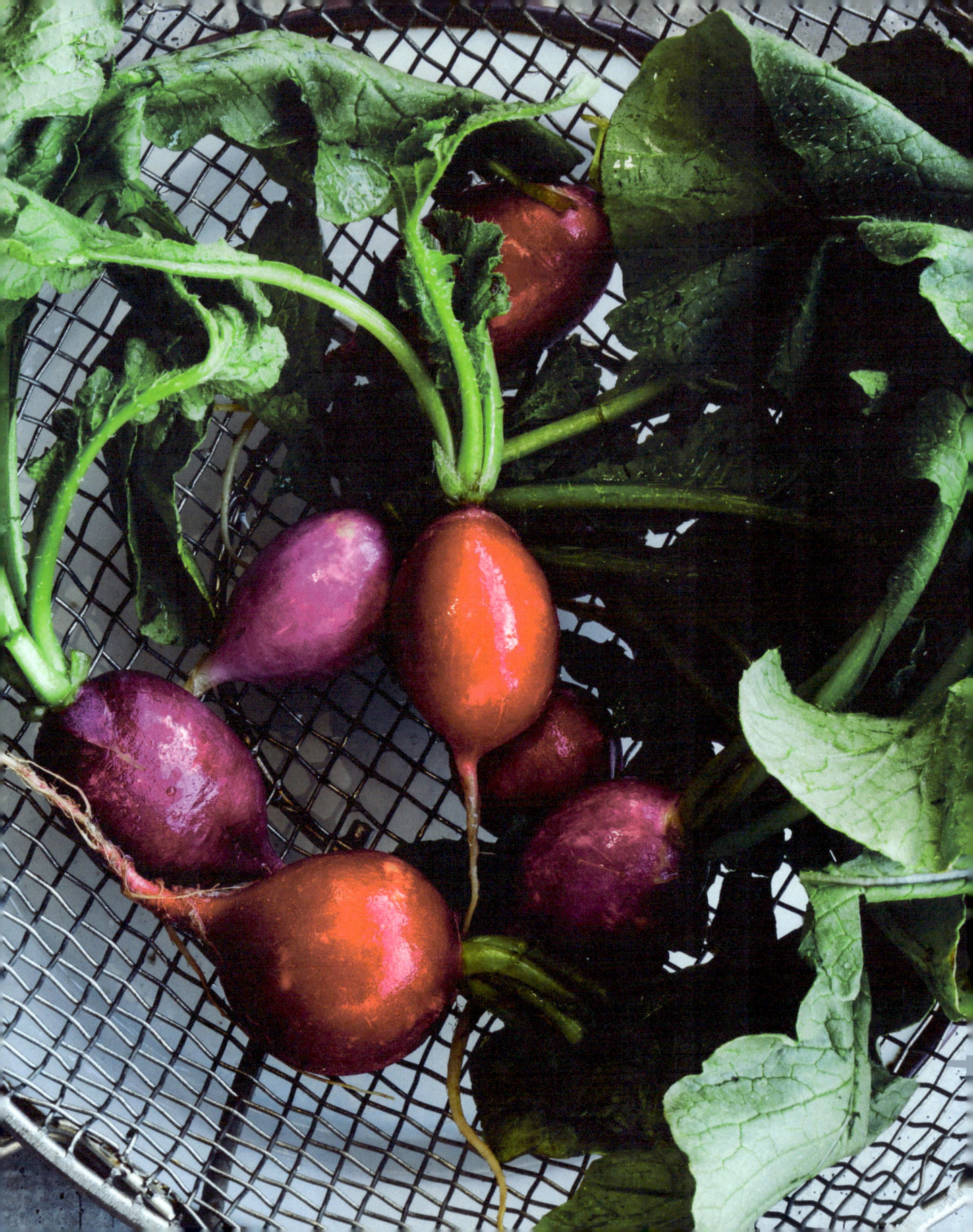

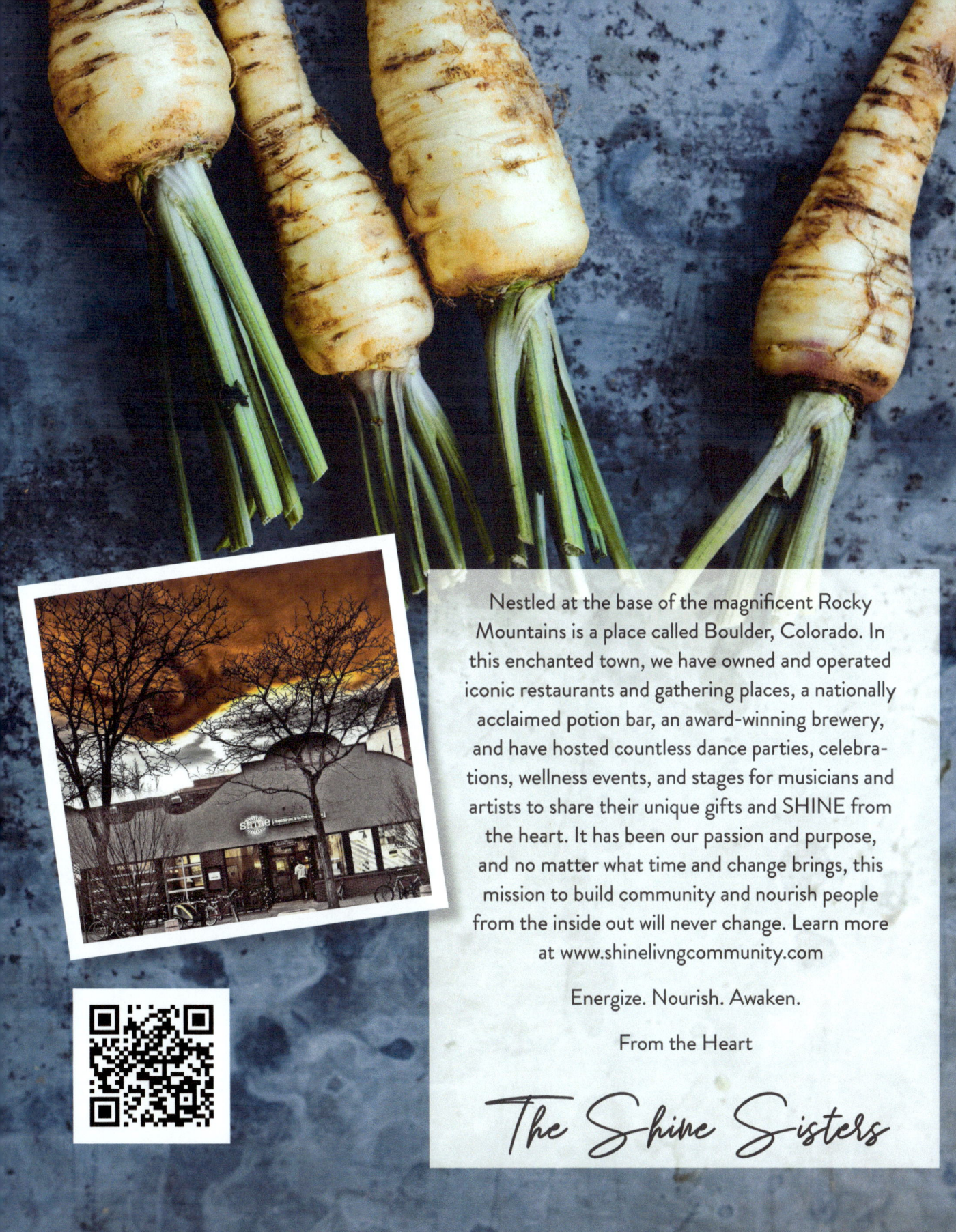

Nestled at the base of the magnificent Rocky Mountains is a place called Boulder, Colorado. In this enchanted town, we have owned and operated iconic restaurants and gathering places, a nationally acclaimed potion bar, an award-winning brewery, and have hosted countless dance parties, celebrations, wellness events, and stages for musicians and artists to share their unique gifts and SHINE from the heart. It has been our passion and purpose, and no matter what time and change brings, this mission to build community and nourish people from the inside out will never change. Learn more at www.shinelivngcommunity.com

Energize. Nourish. Awaken.

From the Heart

The Shine Sisters

INDEX

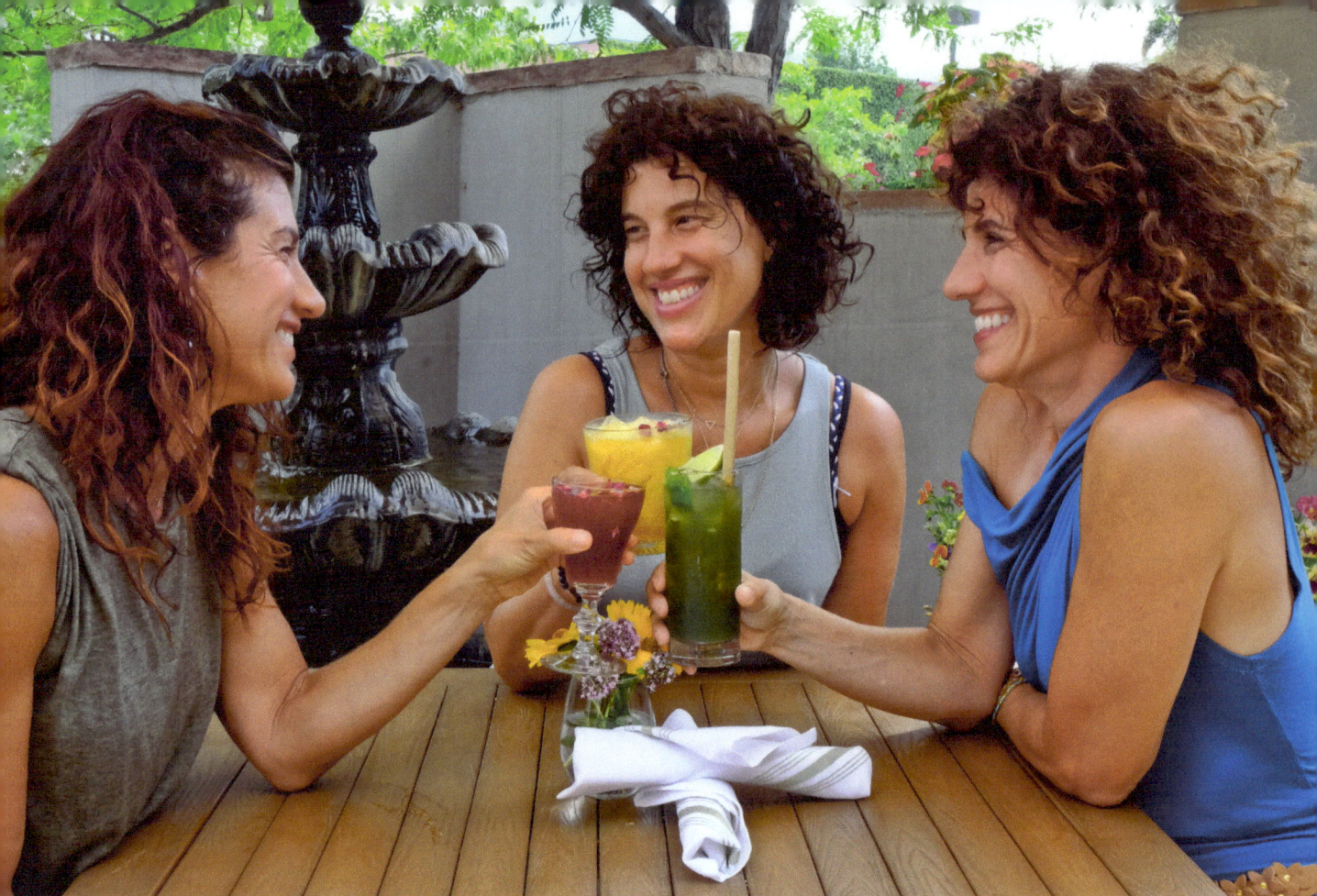

IN DEEP GRATITUDE

From the three of us:

To our publisher, Deborah, and the team at Highlander Press: Thank you for seeing the vision in a second edition of this book and for being a vessel for women's voices to be heard around the globe.

To Eva Kolenko: The badass passionate photographer, who captured our food creations so eloquently.

To Jeffrey Larsen: Our talented food stylist, who took such care and pride in his work to bring our recipes to life.

To Shadi Ramey: Our diligent and fearless recipe tester, who met our crazy for getting the job done in an unbelievably short amount of time.

To Chantal Pierret, founder of Emerging Women and Emerging Human: For that pivotal brainstorming session that was an invitation for us to fully step into our SHINE and OWN it.

To Golden Hoof: For allowing us to use your beautiful farm for our author shots in the first edition, and for being such an inspiration to so many in the way you live and steward the land and animals to provide nourishment for so many.

To Cary Jobe: For our beautiful author shots in the first edition, and for wrangling in and capturing our family and a brand-new puppy down by the Boulder Creek for the second edition author shots.

To our brother Dennis: You have taught us so much about patience, compassion, about how love heals, and we are so much more powerful than we can ever imagine. You are the reason we do the work we do on this planet. You are a gift, and your incredible heart will live with us forever and ever.

To our Mom and Dad, Maureen and Dennis: You have been an incredible guiding light on our path. Thank you for always nurturing our creative spirits and for creating a family of love and support that has been an incredible foundation from which to fly. And mom—our adventures together are the best!

A shout out to our big Italian family: Your wildness and the way you live and love full on and all out,

taught us from a young age to think outside the box and to go after our dreams. That life is not about if you win or lose but rather about the incredible journey, and that love and laughter always prevails.

To our SHINE team from today to the span of twenty-five years: For supporting our hairbrained ideas and for helping bring our visions into reality. We continue to learn so much from each and every one of you.

And to our incredible Shine Living Community: We were built for these times and inspired community is the way forward. The energy we get to create together to transform, heal, and harness joy are such a blessing. Thank you for your willingness, your courage and your commitment to yourself and to this work. Together we RISE and SHINE and SHIMMER the field around us, lighting up the hearts of humanity. Onward we go, step by step.

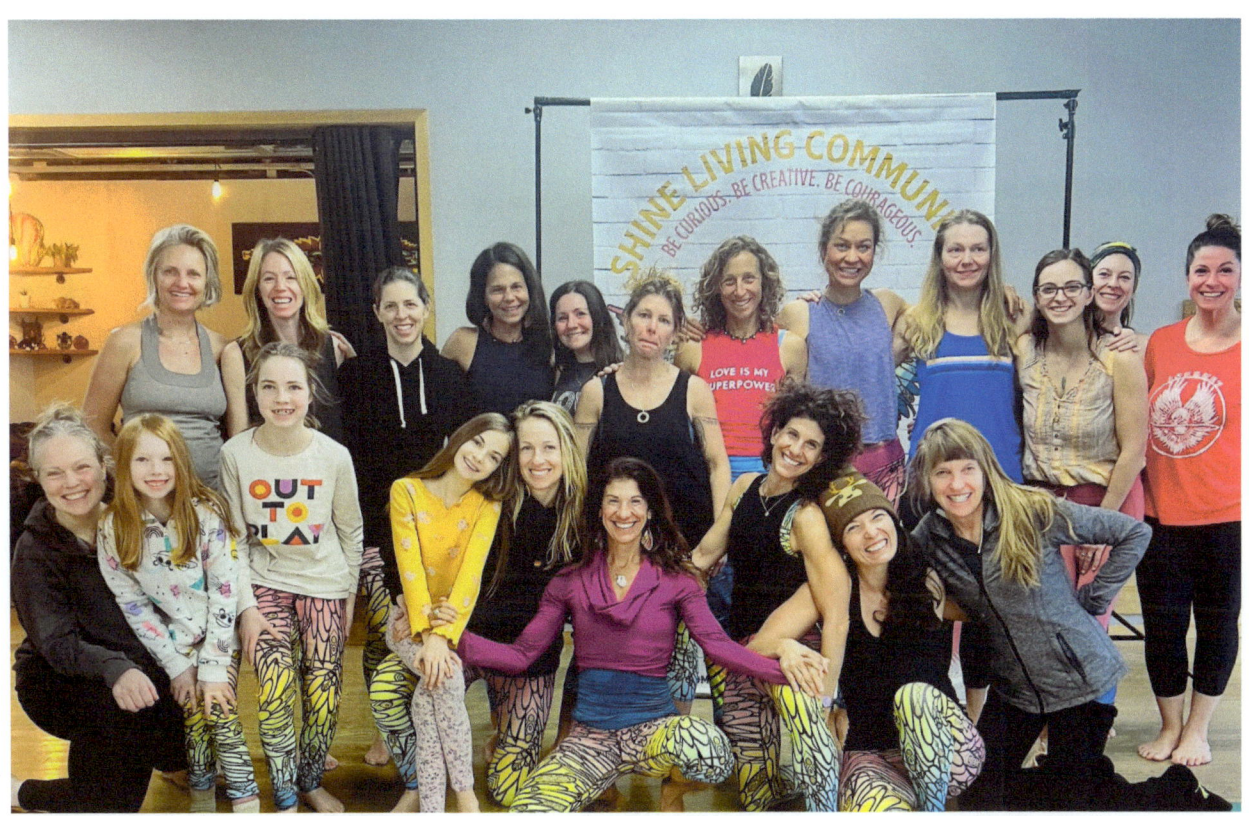

Jessica: To my husband Marek, for teaching me so much about love and partnership. Your kindness, patience and acceptance never cease to amaze me. I feel so blessed to be in this together. To my beautiful daughters, Sofie and Amelie, for bringing out a part of myself I never knew existed—and to introduce me to a love that was beyond my wildest dream. You both inspire me deeply. And to my sisters, who have been my loving support since the womb: you have brought strength and courage to my entire being because I know you are always by my side.

Jill: To my husband Steve, thank you for showing up at exactly the right time and for always believing in me. To my nieces, you remind me of my playful spirit and of how big we can love. You are both incredible

souls and I feel so blessed I get to be your Auntie. To my sisters, my soul mates, I am so happy we chose to walk this path together. You both inspire me so much.

Jennifer: To my hubby Eck who loves me for exactly who I am. Thank you for supporting me to do whatever makes me happy. I feel beyond blessed to share this lifetime with you. And to my nieces, you brighten my every day.

From the heart,

The Shine Sisters

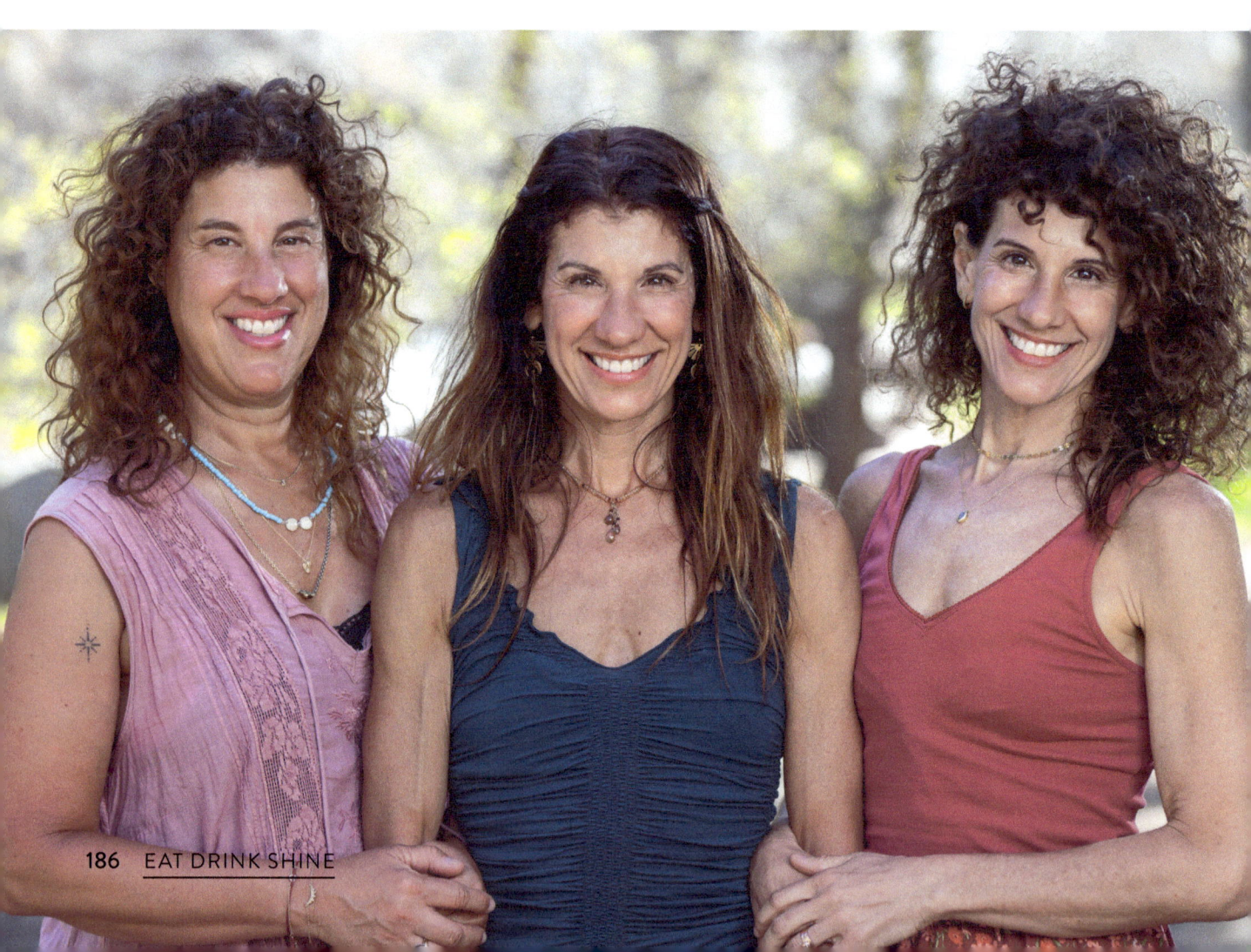

Jessica Emich: First born of triplets and, I like to say, the alpha of the three. I am in awe of how we can access the healer within and transform on every level through food, movement and deep diving into the layers within. I am so grateful it is my life's work to continue to teach and learn about this process. My studies include:

◆ Master's degree in holistic nutrition and graduate of chef instruction from the California Culinary Academy
◆ Certified Yoga Teacher and Breathwork Facilitator and a devoted practitioner for over 25 years
◆ Master Reiki Practitioner

I bring all of my training, personal experience, and loving heart to teach these modalities through SHINE Living Community. As a mother of girls, I understand the importance of practicing in a multigenerational community that inspires each other to keep evolving towards our greatest and most authentic expression of self. You can find me in the mountains, snowboarding or mountain biking or foraging for mushrooms. Or I'll be teaching and practicing at one of our events. I reside in Boulder, Colorado with my husband and our two daughters.

Jill Emich: The middle of the triplet sisters, my mission and purpose in life is to continually encourage people (including myself) to explore and dig deeper into their unique beings, and to share their gifts and passions from the heart. My studies include:

◆ Graduate of hotel restaurant management and culinary arts
◆ Certified dance instructor in an array of modalities
◆ Certified somatic-centered transformation coach/mentor
◆ Certified somatic breathwork Instructor
◆ Movement choreographer and music curator

I passionately blend all of these modalities together and, through science and our own inner wisdom, invite people to get curious, to dissolve old patterns and belief systems, to create a life in joy and authenticity. I live in Boulder, Colorado, with my hubby Steve, our cat Molly, and our dog Daisy. When not practicing and playing with our Shine Living Community, you can find us exploring the world in our camper van, climbing mountains and dancing the night or day away.

Jennifer Emich: The youngest of the three and the most even keeled. I love working with all types of people and learning what uniquely makes them smile. I come from a background of elementary education and always ran the front of house operations at our restaurants. It has taught me to be a great listener and con-nector. I live in Boulder, Colorado, with my husband Eric and our cat Willow. When not practicing real estate, you can find me surrounded by family. I enjoy pickleball, golf, hiking, being with friends, and anything in nature.

"CONNECT TO YOUR HEART, SHINE FROM WITHIN AND THE MAGIC'S IN YOU"

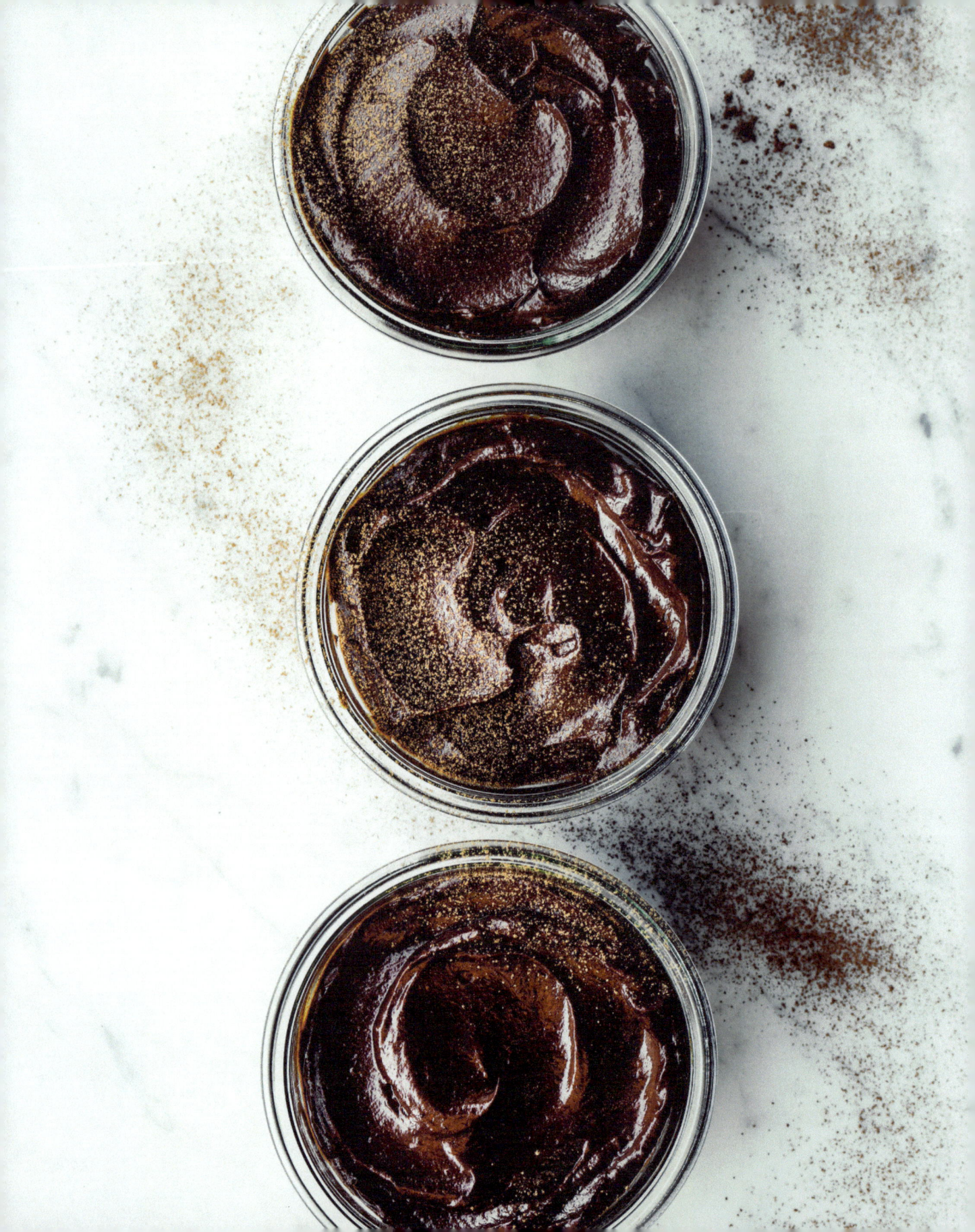